Core Anatomy for Students

Core Anatomy for Students

Other titles also available

Core Anatomy for Students

Volume 1: The Limbs and Vertebral Column

Christopher Dean

*Department of Anatomy and Developmental Biology,
University College London,
London, UK*

and

John Pegington

*Department of Anatomy and Developmental Biology,
University College London,
London, UK*

WB SAUNDERS COMPANY LTD
London   Philadelphia   Toronto   Sydney   Tokyo

W.B. Saunders Company Ltd   24–28 Oval Road
London NW1 7DX, UK

The Curtis Center
Independence Square West
Philadelphia, PA 19106-3399, USA

Harcourt Brace & Company
55 Horner Avenue
Toronto, Ontario M8Z 4X6, Canada

Harcourt Brace & Company, Australia
30–52 Smidmore Street
Marrickville
NSW 2204, Australia

Harcourt Brace & Company, Japan
Ichibancho Central Building
22-1 Ichibancho
Chiyoda-ku, Tokyo 102, Japan

British Library Cataloguing in Publication Data is available from the British Library

ISBN 0-7020-2040-0

Typeset by Photo·graphics, Honiton, Devon.
Printed and bound by The Bath Press, Avon, UK

Core Anatomy for Students is dedicated to the memory of John Pegington. Few people have thought harder about how to teach anatomy for the first time. Few people have been as successful at it.

Contents

Preface

Core Anatomy for Students was written as a revision text. It was originally intended for students who may have left themselves short of time to work for exams, or for those who may be faced with sitting anatomy exams for a second time. We presume, therefore, that students who use one or all of these three volumes will already have completed an anatomy course and will therefore be familiar with basic anatomical terminology. We expect that they will have studied some developmental biology and histology, and also that those who use this text will be keen to start their clinical studies and will be curious to know why a good deal of anatomy is clinically important. With these things in mind we have occasionally drawn freely on developmental anatomy and some applied anatomy in each of these three volumes to clarify or to illustrate what we feel is important material.

These volumes are not designed to be used as a standard textbook or reference book of anatomy. They are meant to provide a framework for revision and self-directed learning. They represent a synopsis of basic material that we feel defines a core of useful knowledge. We regard this core as material that lies in the current mainstream of a continuous learning programme such as medicine. It is that material which we consider as necessary to know in order to understand the next step in this sequence of learning. The content of each volume is highly selective and many things have deliberately been left out. Neither do we intend *Core Anatomy for Students* to be a set of revision *notes* where factual details are maximally condensed. Our emphasis here is on a readable text that explains, sometimes at length, what may be difficult or important. On occasions the text is deliberately repetitious. We have tried to promote an understanding of anatomy in a way that reinforces the learning process, which we feel is not achieved by lists of things to be revised and committed to memory.

The material presented here is probably not set out in a way that parallels the way it was first taught. We hope that the order in which things are presented makes functional and logical sense, and also ties together some topics that may otherwise seem unrelated. Above all, we hope that each section of each volume forms a cogent revision programme in its own right and that dental, medical, speech science, podiatry, physiotherapy and other students who study anatomy will find *Core Anatomy for Students* useful.

Acknowledgements

In the first instance we would like to acknowledge Dr Wojtek Krzemieniewski who drew earlier versions of some of the illustrations we have used. We are especially grateful to Breda O'Connor for typing a great deal of the manuscript and to Dr Deana D'Souza for her scrutiny of the text and illustrations. We are grateful to Barry Johnson and Derek Dudley for technical support and to Jane Pendjiky and Chris Sym for photographic assistance. In particular, we are grateful to many generations of anatomy, dental, medical, speech science, podiatry and physiotherapy students from The School of Medicine, Ottawa, and from University College London, who have all used earlier versions of this revision text, and who over the years have encouraged us to write more of them, to improve them, correct them and finally to publish them. It goes without saying that the artwork in any anatomy book is fundamental to its success. We are especially grateful to Joanna Cameron for her exceptional illustrations. We would also like to express our thanks to the production team at W.B. Saunders, London.

Introduction

Volume 1 of *Core Anatomy For Students* is set out in three sections. The first section covers the upper limb, the second the lower limb and the third the vertebral column. While each of these sections is complete in its own right and can be studied in any order, we suggest the way they are set out may be the most appropriate order to work through them, since occasional reference is made later on to material discussed in the earlier sections.

We have made no attempt to reduce the chapters in each volume to an equal length. As they stand they represent what we feel are coherent functional units which all form part of a sequential revision programme. The illustrations are for the most part designed to be coloured in as you work through the text. We would encourage you at least to choose a few key diagrams in each section to colour in, since there is evidence that this helps to commit the three-dimensional aspects of anatomy to memory. The legends for each diagram can also be used as a summary of the text when revising each section on subsequent occasions.

At the end of each section there is a revision chapter to help consolidate your anatomical knowledge and to test your understanding of each region. You may choose to do the multiple choice questions a few at a time as you finish reading each chapter. You may prefer to do them all together at the end of each section. Alternatively, you might even consider doing the even-numbered questions on your first attempt and the odd-numbered questions on a subsequent occasion. Whatever you decide, remember that they are an integral part of this revision programme and that you need to work through them with reference to the text at some stage to get the most out of your revision. Do not be tempted to ignore them altogether.

THE UPPER LIMB

The Shoulder

The focal point of the shoulder region is the shoulder joint. All of the structures around the joint are arranged so that this widely mobile articulation can place the upper limb in a wide variety of positions. The joint is clothed with muscles on all sides, except below. In front are the two flat **pectoral muscles** (Fig. 1.1). This area can therefore be called the **pectoral region**. Behind the joint there are also muscles that sandwich a plate of bone called the **scapula** between them. These muscles together with the scapula form the **scapular region** (Fig. 1.2). A cape of muscle called the **deltoid** drapes over the top of the joint between these two regions, so forming another region above them that we can call the **deltoid region** (Fig. 1.2).

The muscle groups, both anterior and posterior to the shoulder joint, form two walls of a pyramidal space that lies between the upper arm and the chest wall. This space is called the armpit or **axilla**. The pectoral region, therefore, takes part in the formation of the **anterior wall of the axilla** and the scapular region in the formation of the **posterior wall**. The **medial wall** is

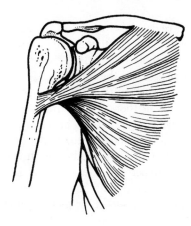

Figure 1.1 The pectoral muscles take part in the formation of the anterior wall of the axilla. Pectoralis major is shown here.

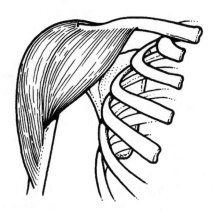
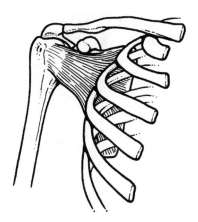

Figure 1.2 The scapula and subscapularis muscle with the deltoid muscle above.

of course the chest wall itself. A large muscle called the **serratus anterior** lies over this wall of the axilla.

The nerve plexus for the upper limb is derived from **ventral rami** whose segmental origin is almost completely from the neck. This plexus streams over the first rib into the axilla. It is called the **brachial plexus**. Journeying with the nerves is an artery, a vein and some lymphatics. These structures together may be said to constitute the contents of the axilla.

A logical plan of study is therefore to look first at the regions defined above, the pectoral, scapular, deltoid and serratus anterior regions, because these define the boundaries of the axilla. The axillary contents can then be studied and finally the shoulder joint itself can be described.

The pectoral region

The pectoral region lies in front of the shoulder joint and chest wall. If the soft tissues are removed, its bony framework is visible (Fig. 1.3). Three bones need to be identified. These are the **humerus**, the **scapula** and the **clavicle**. Do not try to study them separately but rather arranged in their normal anatomical position with their normal articulations apparent.

The humerus is the bone of the upper arm but only its proximal part need be studied with the pectoral region. At the upper end is a spherical **head**, which during life is covered with articular cartilage. The head fits against the socket, or **glenoid cavity**, of the

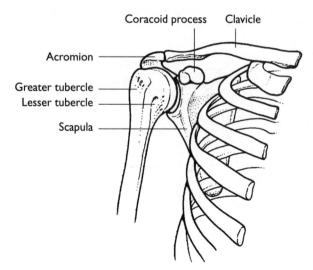

Figure 1.3   The humerus, clavicle and scapula.

Labels on figure:
Coracoid process   Clavicle
Acromion
Greater tubercle
Lesser tubercle
Scapula

scapula to form the shoulder joint. The head of the humerus is set on a very stout **anatomical neck**.

Two bony prominences are easily identified just distal to the head and neck. These are the **greater** and **lesser tubercles**. They arise during development and are associated with muscles that pull on the proximal end of the humerus. In fact several of the shoulder muscles insert into this region of the humerus. The tubercles can be traced down the humerus for a short way as two raised ridges. These bony ridges are called the **crests** of the greater and lesser tubercles. A groove is formed between the tubercles and their corresponding crests. This is called the **intertubercular groove**.

Below the head, neck, tubercles and crests of the humerus the shaft of the bone narrows. It is at this point that the bone sometimes breaks. This area is therefore sometimes referred to as the **surgical neck of the humerus** to distinguish it from the anatomical neck that we described above. A little further distally the outer aspect of the shaft of the humerus is raised into an roughened area called the **deltoid tuberosity**. This marks the region into which the cape-like deltoid muscle is inserted.

The scapula resembles a triangular plate of bone, applied to the side and back of the chest wall. Most of it is hidden from view in Figure 1.3. The lateral edge of the plate can be seen and, at the upper end of this, the **glenoid cavity** faces outwards to accommodate the head of the humerus. The glenoid is covered with articular cartilage. A beak-like process of the scapula can also be identified projecting forwards; this is the **coracoid process**. A second process can also be seen projecting from the back of the plate. This is the **acromion** and it articulates with the lateral end of the clavicle.

The clavicle describes a gentle 'S-shaped' curve from the acromion towards the midline of the body. It is subcutaneous and therefore easily palpated. Its lateral end articulates with the acromion at the **acromioclavicular joint**. The medial end articulates with the part of the sternum called the manubrium at the **sternoclavicular joint**. This latter joint is the only true **articulation** between the trunk and the pectoral girdle besides attachments through ligaments and muscles. Both the acromioclavicular and sternoclavicular joints are synovial. Now identify the same bony landmarks on a radiograph of the shoulder (Fig. 1.4).

To complete the study of the pectoral region we need to describe the muscles and their deep fascia which attach to the bones of the pectoral girdle. There

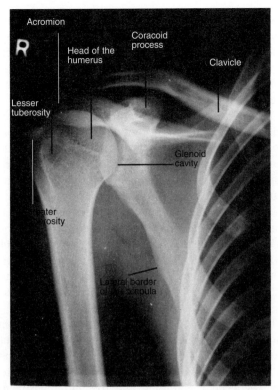

Figure 1.4 Anteroposterior radiograph of the shoulder region.

are in fact two layers of muscle: a deeper layer consisting of the **pectoralis minor** and **subclavius** (Fig. 1.5) and a more massive superficial layer composed of the **pectoralis major**.

The pectoralis minor is triangular in shape. The base of this triangular muscle forms its origin. It arises from the middle three true ribs on the front of the chest. The apex of the muscle inserts on to the coracoid process. When it contracts, the pectoralis minor draws the process downwards, thus depressing the shoulder. However, if the scapula is fixed by stabilizing the pectoral girdle, then the origin and insertion switch round. In this situation the pectoralis minor may act as an accessory muscle of respiration and raise the rib cage. This can often be seen when patients with chronic lung disease hold on to the side of the bed or bed table, or simply fix their hands on their hips, in order to be able to use this muscle to aid breathing.

The subclavius is a small muscle arising from the upper surface of the first rib. Its fibres slope upwards and laterally to be inserted into the under-surface of the clavicle. The muscle has a steadying action on the clavicle during shoulder movements. The first rib and manubrium form an immobile primary cartilaginous joint. It is on this immobile 'platform' that the medial end of the clavicle pivots (Fig. 1.6). It is not surprising, therefore, to find such a strong muscle and also strong ligaments anchored to this region. The deep fascia and periosteum that cover the clavicle run off it to enclose the pectoralis minor muscle beneath. This loose connective tissue is called the **clavipectoral fascia**.

The pectoralis major (Fig. 1.7) is a powerful muscle which extends from the front of the chest to the humerus. It takes origin superficial to the pectoralis minor, subclavius and clavipectoral fascia. Part of the muscle takes origin from the front of the medial half of the clavicle and part from the front of the sternum, upper costal cartilages and external oblique aponeurosis. The two portions are divided by a deep cleft. As the muscle fibres pass to their insertion into the crest of the greater tubercle of the humerus (Fig. 1.1), they twist, the lowest fibres sweeping up to insert behind

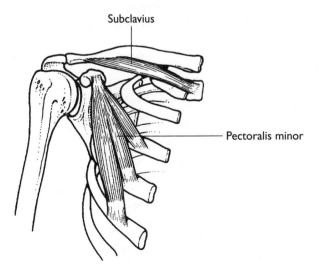

Figure 1.5 The pectoralis minor and subclavius muscles.

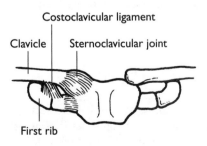

Figure 1.6 The first rib, manubrium and clavicle.

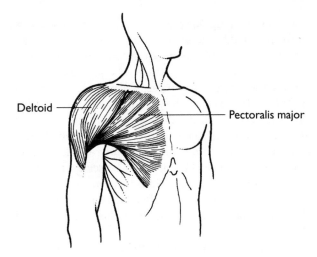

Figure 1.7   Pectoralis major.

the clavicular fibres. It is this arrangement that gives the rounded, full appearance to the lower border of the muscle, which in turn underlies the appearance of the anterior axillary fold.

The pectoralis major is a powerful *adductor* of the upper limb. It can also medially rotate the arm. The deep fascia on the surface of the muscle is strong and, in the female, forms the base on which the breast rests. A deeply seated cancer of the breast may invade the fascia and eventually the muscle. It is therefore important to be able to test the action of the muscle in such patients in order to determine whether or not such a cancer has become fixed to the muscle. This can be done by asking the patient to press both hands on her hips. In this situation the muscle is tense and any lump in the breast can now be tested for mobility. If it remains fixed during this test it provides evidence that the spreading cancer has already infiltrated the underlying deep fascia and muscle.

The pectoral region defines the **anterior wall of the axilla**. This wall is made up of the **pectoralis minor**, **subclavius** and **clavipectoral fascia** on a deep plane, and the **pectoralis major** with its **fascia** more superficially.

The scapular region

The bony scapula is suspended in place against the back of the chest wall by muscles that attach it to the trunk and by ligaments that attach it to the clavicle. The scapula is therefore mobile. We have already described most of the bony landmarks on the scapula. However, note also that its upper border is notched. The **scapular notch** allows an important neurovascular bundle to reach the muscles on the back of the bone. The large flat surface of the scapula seen from the front is called the **subscapular fossa**.

Viewed from the front, two muscles can be seen arising from the scapula (one from in front and one from behind) and passing laterally to insert into the humerus. They are the **subscapularis** and the **teres major** (Fig. 1.8). The subscapularis muscle is a thick muscular mass arising from the subscapular fossa. It is a multipennate muscle and therefore capable of long and sustained contraction. The fibres converge to form a tendon which inserts into the lesser tubercle of the humerus. As this tendon passes over the front to the shoulder joint some of its fibres blend and fuse with the capsule of the joint. The muscle is an *adductor* and *medial rotator* of the humerus.

Usually, there is a hole in the capsule of the shoulder joint in front which allows the **subscapular bursa** to protrude from the joint cavity. This is simply a 'balloon' of synovial membrane which insinuates itself between the muscle and the joint capsule to reduce friction during movement.

The **teres major** is a thick, round muscle arising from the lateral border of the *posterior* surface of the scapular blade. It is inserted in line with and beneath the subscapularis into the crest of the lesser tubercle. Its action is therefore similar to that of the subscapularis. Both muscles also have another important function, that of assisting to maintain the head of the humerus in the glenoid cavity.

Now is a good time to look at a large, flat muscle

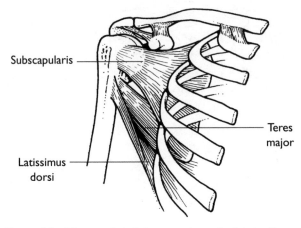

Figure 1.8   The muscles of the posterior wall of the axilla.

on the back of the trunk. This muscle, the **latissimus dorsi**, is part of the external body wall musculature of the trunk but its insertion is into the humerus and therefore it is functionally an 'upper limb' muscle (Fig. 1.9).

The muscle arises from the lower thoracic and lumbar spinous processes and their interspinous ligaments, the thoracolumbar fascia and the iliac crest. From this wide area its fibres sweep up towards the lower angle of the scapula and then onwards to insert by means of a strong, flat tendon into the intertubercular groove of the humerus. In so doing, it skirts the lower border of teres major (Fig. 1.9). The latissimus dorsi is the great climbing muscle. It *adducts* and *medially rotates* the humerus. In climbing, with the hands gripping a fixed point above, the muscle draws the whole trunk upwards.

We can now define the **posterior wall of the axilla**. It is formed by the **subscapularis** and the **teres major** with the **tendon of the latissimus dorsi** winding around the lower border of the teres major. The rounded appearance of the posterior wall is called the **posterior fold** of the axilla and comes about because of this relationship between latissimus dorsi and teres major.

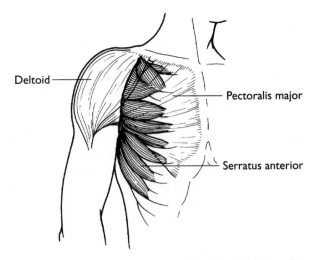

Figure 1.10 Serratus anterior on the medial wall of the axilla.

The serratus anterior

The serratus anterior (Fig. 1.10) lies against the side of the chest wall. It is a flat muscle, arranged in slips or digitations, and it holds the medial border of the scapula against the chest wall. It also aids in rotatory movements of the scapula on the chest wall. Together with the upper ribs, it forms the **medial wall of the axilla**. The digitations arise from the first eight ribs and then curve back around the side of the chest wall to gain insertion into the *medial* margin of the scapula. The muscle can therefore pull the scapula forwards around the chest wall, an action called **protraction** (Fig. 1.11).

The muscle has a further action in that it holds the

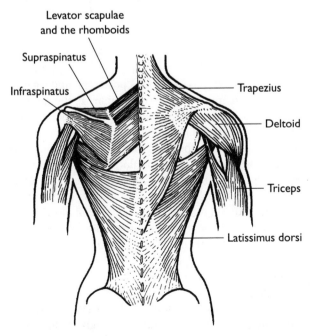

Figure 1.9 Muscles of the back that act on the scapula or humerus.

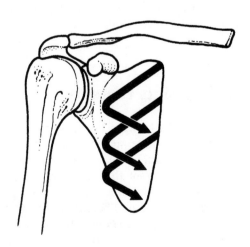

Figure 1.11 Protraction is brought about by serratus anterior.

medial edge of the scapula close against the chest wall. If it is paralysed, the medial border of the scapula splays out from its bed. This condition is occasionally found after operations for carcinoma of the breast in which there have been injuries to the nerve supply of the muscle. The condition is called a 'winged scapula'. The muscle also helps in rotation of the scapula on the chest wall. It does this especially by means of its lowermost fibres which rotate the scapula so that the glenoid faces upwards. If the pectoral girdle is fixed, the muscle can, like the pectoral muscles, also act as an accessory muscle of respiration.

The deltoid region

The deltoid is a powerful, triangular cape of muscle covering the shoulder (Figs 1.9 and 1.10). It is another multipennate muscle and therefore capable of long sustained action. It has a 'U-shaped' origin when viewed from above, which runs from the outer margins of the lateral part of the clavicle, across the acromion and then on to the spine of the scapula. The muscle narrows to pass laterally from this line of origin towards the shaft of the humerus. It is inserted on to the deltoid tuberosity of the humerus. A large bursa separates the undersurface of the muscle from the underlying shoulder joint to prevent friction here. This bursa is called the **subacromial bursa** and will be described in more detail later.

The deltoid is a very versatile muscle, its anterior fibres, acting alone, can flex the arm and the posterior fibres reverse this movement and extend the arm. The fibres in the middle, that directly overlie the shoulder joint, make up the chief *abductor* muscle of the arm at the shoulder joint.

The axilla and its contents

The pyramidal cavity between the upper arm and the chest wall is called the armpit or **axilla**. The apex of this pyramid lies medial to the coracoid process of the scapula. It is at this point that structures enter and leave the upper limb. The entrance is bounded by the clavicle in front, the outer border of the first rib medially, and the upper margin of the scapula posteriorly (Figs 1.12 and 1.13). The walls of the axilla have already been studied.

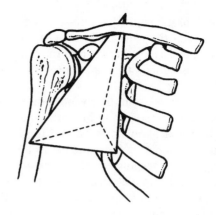

Figure 1.12   The boundaries of the axilla are three walls and a base.

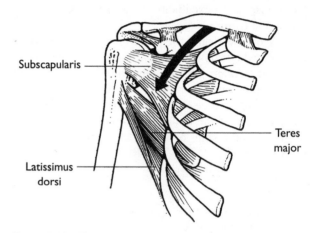

Figure 1.13   The entrance to the axilla.

The pyramid has **anterior**, **posterior** and **medial walls**, a **base** and an **apex**. To summarize, the **anterior wall** is made up of the **pectoralis minor**, **subclavius** and **clavipectoral fascia** deeply, and the **pectoralis major** on a more superficial plane. The **posterior wall** is composed of the **subscapularis** and **teres major**, with the **latissimus tendon** winding around its lower border. The anterior and posterior folds of the axilla are rounded and curved. The **medial wall of the axilla** is formed by the **serratus anterior** and the upper ribs that lie deep to this muscle. The base of the axilla is the skin of the armpit. Running through the axilla are several structures. First, the plexus of nerves to the upper limb arises in the neck. It is called the **brachial plexus** and many of the nerves that arise from the plexus enter the axilla through the apex and are then distributed as terminal branches to the limb.

The **axillary artery** is a continuation of the subclavian artery. This enters by the same route as the brachial plexus, and is the arterial supply to the limb. The **axillary vein** accompanies the artery on its way to the root of the neck, where it is renamed the subclavian vein. Arranged around the vascular structures in the axilla are several important groups of lymph nodes.

The brachial plexus

The nerve supply to the upper limb is derived from the ventral rami of the 5th, 6th, 7th and 8th cervical spinal nerves and part of the ventral ramus of the 1st thoracic spinal nerve. The ventral rami emerge from between the scalenus anterior and medius in the neck (Fig. 1.14). Here they immediately enter the so-called **posterior triangle** of the neck. This triangle is outlined by the sternocleidomastoid muscle, the clavicle and the trapezius. (Define it on Figure 1.14.) It is here, in the posterior triangle, that the six ventral rami fuse to form three **trunks** (Fig. 1.15). The 5th and 6th cervical ventral rami fuse to form the **upper trunk**. The 7th cervical ventral ramus remains free as the **middle trunk** and the 8th cervical and 1st thoracic ventral rami fuse as the **lower trunk**.

At this level in the brachial plexus four branches are given off (Fig. 1.16). Two of these go to scapular muscles on the back. One goes to the subclavius and the other to the serratus anterior. The nerves to the

scapular muscles are called the **dorsal scapular** and **suprascapular nerves**. The **dorsal scapular nerve** passes back between the muscles in the depths of the posterior triangle to reach the levator scapulae and

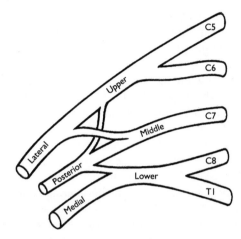

Figure 1.15 The six ventral rami of the brachial plexus fuse to form three trunks.

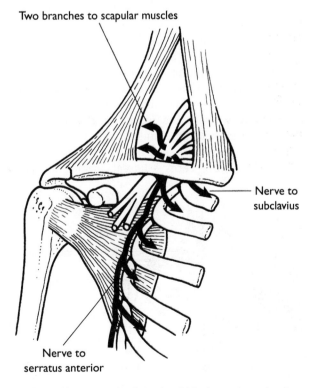

Figure 1.16 Branches of the brachial plexus that arise from the trunks.

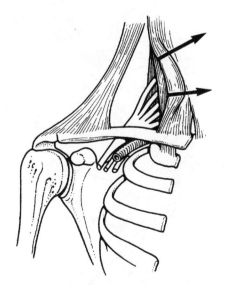

Figure 1.14 The ventral rami of the brachial plexus can be seen emerging between scalenus medius and scalenus anterior in the posterior triangle of the neck.

rhomboids (Fig. 1.17). The **suprascapular nerve** also passes back, aiming for the scapular notch on the upper border of the scapula. It passes on to the back of the scapula to supply the two muscles covering the posterior surface of this bone (supraspinatus and infraspinatus, which we will study shortly). This is illustrated in Figure 1.17. The **nerve to subclavius** descends in front of the plexus to reach the deep surface of the muscle. The **long thoracic nerve** descends over the surface of the serratus anterior, supplying this muscle along its course. As its name implies it is a fairly long nerve and, as it lies on the medial wall of the axilla, it is vulnerable during operations for carcinoma of the breast.

A short distance *behind* the clavicle, each of these trunks divides into **anterior** and **posterior divisions**. These divisions then unite in such a way that **three cords** are formed. They are the **lateral, medial** and **posterior** cords (Fig. 1.15). The cords lie in the axilla arranged around the axillary artery. In fact they are named according to their relationship to the axillary artery. The lateral and medial cords are destined to supply all the **flexor aspects** of the limb and the posterior cord the **extensor aspects** (Fig. 1.18).

To summarize so far look at Figure 1.19 and trace through the formation of the brachial plexus. (1) The brachial plexus is formed from the ventral rami of C5, 6, 7 and 8, and T1. These come into view between the scalenus anterior and scalenus medius. (2) In the posterior triangle of the neck these ventral rami unite to form upper, middle and lower trunks. Four branches arise from the plexus at this point. (3) Behind the clavicle the trunks divide into divisions which then reunite in such a way as to form three cords. These three cords – lateral, medial and pos-

terior – are arranged around the axillary artery in the axilla (4).

Now trace the terminal branches from the lateral and medial cords (Fig. 1.20). These are destined to supply the flexor aspect of the limb (both muscles and sensation).

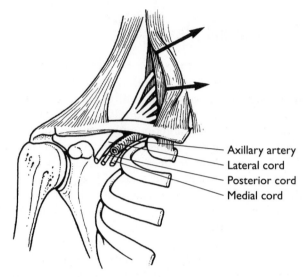

Axillary artery
Lateral cord
Posterior cord
Medial cord

Figure 1.18 The lateral, posterior and medial cords of the brachial plexus arranged around the axillary artery.

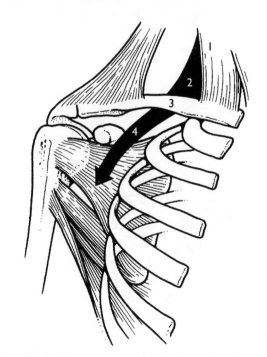

Figure 1.19 Diagram summarizing the formation of the brachial plexus.

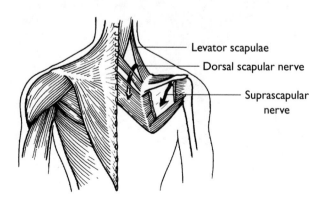

Levator scapulae
Dorsal scapular nerve
Suprascapular nerve

Figure 1.17 Nerves to the scapular muscles.

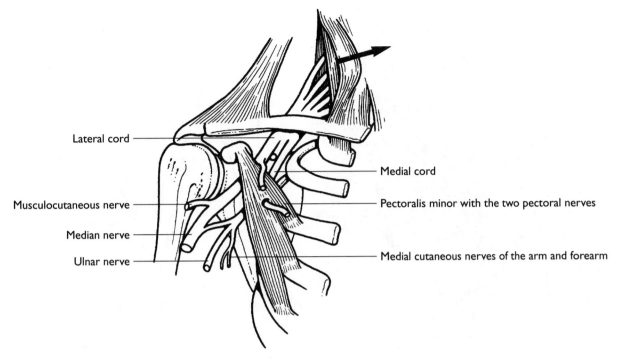

Lateral cord

Musculocutaneous nerve

Median nerve

Ulnar nerve

Medial cord

Pectoralis minor with the two pectoral nerves

Medial cutaneous nerves of the arm and forearm

Figure 1.20   Terminal branches of the lateral and medial cords of the brachial plexus.

The pectoral nerves

The lateral and medial pectoral nerves arise from the lateral and medial cords respectively (which is how they get their names). The lateral pectoral nerve pierces the clavipectoral fascia and then enters the pectoralis major. The medial nerve enters the deep surface of the pectoralis minor. Some of its fibres pass right through this muscle and aid in the supply of the pectoralis major as well.

The musculocutaneous nerve

This nerve arises from the lateral cord and passes immediately into the combined muscle mass of biceps and coracobrachialis. The lateral cord then continues on as the **median nerve**. The median nerve is the continuation of the lateral cord, but it also receives a contribution from the medial cord. It is concerned with much of the supply to the flexor aspect of the arm below the elbow.

The ulnar nerve

The ulnar nerve is the continuation of the medial cord and also supplies flexor aspects below the elbow. Also arising from the medial cord are two cutaneous nerves, the **medial cutaneous nerve of arm** and the **medial cutaneous nerve of forearm**. Figure 1.20 shows the lateral and medial cords with their terminal branches. The posterior cord in this diagram has been cut in the axilla to make their relationships easier to follow. Figure 1.21 illustrates the posterior cord and its terminal branches, and in this diagram the lateral and medial cords have been cut in the axilla to simplify the picture. The **posterior cord** gives terminal branches which go to the extensor aspects of the limb (Fig. 1.21). The **subscapular nerves** and the **thoracodorsal** nerve supply the muscles of the **posterior wall of the axilla**. The subscapular nerves supply the subscapularis and the teres major, and the thoracodorsal the latissimus dorsi. The **axillary nerve** passes between the subscapularis and the teres major and then curls round the back of the humerus. Here it lies deep to the deltoid muscle, which it supplies. The

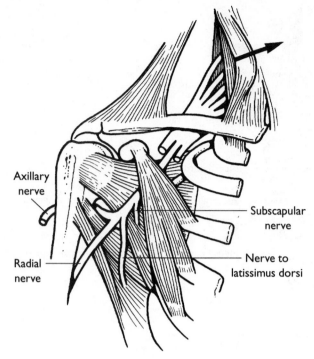

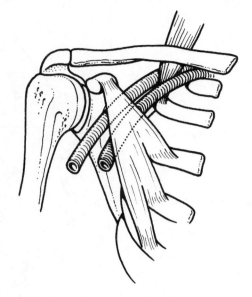

Figure 1.22   The axillary artery and axillary vein.

Figure 1.21   Terminal branches of the posterior cord of the brachial plexus.

posterior cord continues on as the **radial nerve**. This descends to the extensor aspect of the humerus.

The axillary artery and axillary vein

The arterial supply for the upper limb comes from the axillary artery. This is none other than a continuation of the subclavian artery beyond the first rib (Fig. 1.22). The artery enters the axilla through the apex and leaves at the lower border of the teres major where it is then renamed the brachial artery.

The first section of the axillary artery lies deep to the clavipectoral fascia. The next part is deep to the pectoralis minor (Fig. 1.22). As we have seen, the cords of the brachial plexus are arranged around the artery, the lateral cord lying lateral to it, the medial on the medial side and the posterior behind the vessel (Fig. 1.23). The axillary vein lies on the medial side of the neurovascular complex. The lower part of the artery, below the level of pectoralis minor, is surrounded by the terminal branches of the three cords of the brachial plexus (Fig. 1.23).

Notice the arrangement of the branches of the

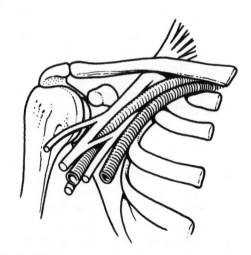

Figure 1.23   The cords of the brachial plexus arranged around the axillary artery.

cords around the artery and vein. The contribution to the median nerve from the medial cord crosses *in front* of the artery. The terminal branches of the medial and lateral cords, the ulnar and median nerves, are seen on either side of the artery. Behind the artery is the posterior cord with its branches.

To find your way around a specimen of the axilla always follow the following procedure. Retract the biceps and coracobrachialis muscles. You will then see the musculocutaneous nerve as it enters them. Trace this nerve back and it will lead you to the lateral cord. The lateral cord traced distally becomes the median nerve. Pull on this median nerve and find the contribution from the medial cord. Traced back, this contribution leads you to the medial cord. Follow the medial cord distally as the ulnar nerve. You have traced a network shaped like a letter 'M'. Follow this procedure on an anatomical specimen several times and you will find identification of the terminal branches of the lateral and medial cords easy.

Like so many other vessels, the branches of the axillary artery are variable. It may be said as a general rule that it is more important for students to learn the *nerves* in the limb than the arterial branches. The branches of the axillary artery supply blood to the scapular muscles and the chest wall and female breast (Fig. 1.24).

The **superior thoracic** branch is small and with the **lateral thoracic** branch and **thoracoacromial** branch supplies much of the muscles, fat and breast on the front of the chest. In the female the lateral thoracic branch is especially large and supplies the breast. Two **circumflex humeral** branches form a vascular arrangement around the surgical neck of the humerus. The posterior one in fact accompanies the axillary nerve to the back of the humerus. The **subscapular artery** accompanies the thoracodorsal nerve. It supplies the subscapularis and teres major with blood and also sends branches into the latissimus dorsi. A circumflex scapular branch arises from it and helps to supply the scapular muscles on the back of that bone.

The scapular muscles receive a good blood supply from the branches of the axillary artery; however, they also receive some blood from the subclavian artery in the root of the neck. These branches cross the posterior triangle and accompany the two branches of the brachial plexus that supply the posterior scapular muscles. Thus, if for any reason there should be a blockage in the first part of the axillary artery, a bypass may develop through this scapular network of vessels. This can sometimes be sufficient to maintain a viable blood supply to the limb. The formation of the **axillary vein** will be described below when the whole venous pattern of the limb is discussed. In the axilla it lies medial to the artery and continues over the upper surface of the first rib, where it is then called the subclavian vein.

Axillary lymph nodes and lymphatics

The lymph nodes in the axilla can be divided into three groups (Fig. 1.25). The **lateral group** lies laterally along the axillary vessels. They receive lymph from the upper limb lymphatics. The **pectoral** or **anterior group** lies anteriorly between the anterior and medial walls of the axilla. The upper nodes of this group lie in the main pathway of lymph coming from the breast. The remainder receive lymph from the side wall of the thorax. The **subscapular** or **posterior group** lies on the posterior wall of the axilla along the sub-

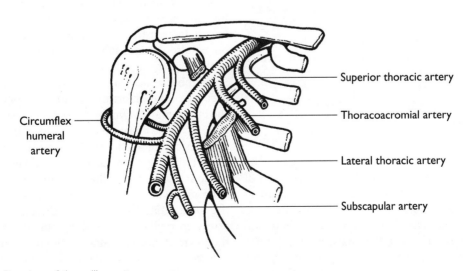

Circumflex humeral artery

Superior thoracic artery

Thoracoacromial artery

Lateral thoracic artery

Subscapular artery

Figure 1.24 Branches of the axillary artery.

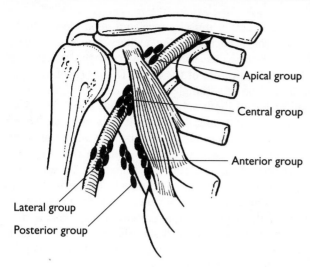

Apical group

Central group

Anterior group

Lateral group

Posterior group

Figure 1.25   The distribution of lymph nodes in the axilla.

scapular vessels. They receive lymph from the scapular region and back. All three groups connect with **central nodes** which lie in the fat of the axilla. Lymph drains eventually from all of the above nodes into the **apical nodes** at the apex of the axilla. The efferents from these form the **subclavian lymph trunk** which usually empties into the subclavian vein. There are a few outlying nodes in the **pectoral region** which, although strictly not 'axillary', should be considered now since they drain into the apical nodes. These include the **infraclavicular nodes**, which lie on the clavipectoral fascia and in the groove between the deltoid and pectoralis major. Although the upper limb lymph drains through the axillary nodes, perhaps more important from a clinical point of view is the fact that much of the lymph from the breast also drains through them. Carcinoma of the breast may spread along these lymphatics and may often involve nodes in the axilla.

The breast

The breast is a glandular structure that lies in the fat of the pectoral region. The gland is larger and of functional importance, of course, in the female. Unfortunately it is also important clinically for another reason: it is often the seat of carcinoma. The lymphatic drainage we have just described must be noted carefully since this is the usual route by which cancer spreads to more distant parts of the body. In the male,

the gland is small and functionless and rarely the seat of cancer. In the female, however, the gland is large and the glandular tissue is embedded in fat. While the breast is producing milk the glandular part enlarges much more than the fatty part of the breast. The gland has no fibrous capsule and this renders direct spread of a cancer to the underlying pectoral muscles a relatively easy matter. The 'base' of the breast rests on the deep fascia of the pectoralis major. It extends from the side of the sternum to the edge of the pectoralis major. Some glandular tissue extends beyond the edge of the muscle to lie on the medial wall of the axilla. An extension reaches high into the axilla and is called the **axillary tail** of the breast.

Above, the breast extends to the second rib and below to the sixth; here at its lower extremity it lies on the origin of the external oblique muscle. Surmounting the breast is the **nipple** and this is surrounded by a circle of dark-coloured skin called the **areolar**. The colour of the nipple and the areolar darkens during the first pregnancy and remains darker thereafter. The glandular tissue itself is divided by **fibrous septa** which pass through the fat from skin to pectoral fascia. The divisions of the gland are called **lobes**. There are usually about 15 or more lobes in each breast. The lobes are further divided into lobules. The milk produced in each lobe is passed towards the nipple through a **lactiferous duct**. Just beneath the nipple each duct expands to form a **lactiferous sinus** before opening on to the nipple (Fig. 1.26).

The blood supply to the breast comes from the **perforating branches** of the **internal thoracic artery** (Fig. 1.27). In the female the branches that pass out into the breast tissue through the second, third and fourth intercostal spaces are particularly large. The breast also receives blood from the thoracic branches of the axillary artery (Fig. 1.24).

Lymphatic drainage of the breast is important because of the unfortunate frequency of carcinoma of the breast and its lymphatic spread. Most of the lymph goes to the **axillary nodes**. Spread of cancer to these nodes becomes apparent as a hard lump in the axilla. (No clinical examination of the breast is complete without feeling the axilla for lumps.)

From the deep parts of the gland lymphatics follow the perforating branches of the internal thoracic artery to nodes that lie along this vessel. These are the **internal thoracic nodes**. From here the lymphatics follow the intercostal artery back to the region of the aorta where they drain into **para-aortic nodes**. In this

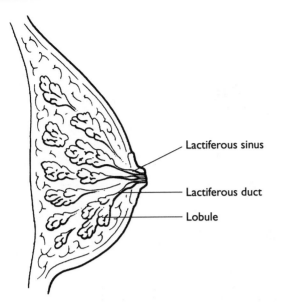

Figure 1.26 Lobules, lactiferous ducts and lactiferous sinuses of the breast.

Lactiferous sinus
Lactiferous duct
Lobule

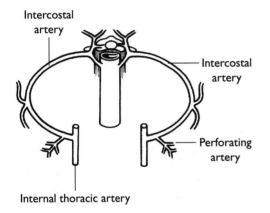

Figure 1.27 The perforating branches of the internal thoracic artery.

Intercostal artery
Intercostal artery
Perforating artery
Internal thoracic artery

way cancer can spread from the breast into the thoracic cavity. Some lymph from the lower part of the gland flows downwards through the abdominal wall, and spread through these lymphatics can take cancer cells into the abdominal cavity. There are some connections between **skin lymphatics** across the midline of the body. Breast cancer sometimes spreads from one breast to the other breast, possibly by this route. Lymph from the nipple and areolar drains into a lymphatic plexus just deep to the surface, called the subareolar plexus. Eventually this drains to the axillary nodes.

Muscles on the back of the scapula

This is a convenient point at which to study a group of muscles on the posterior surface of the scapula and which help to suspend the scapula from the vertebral column. This will complete our study of the muscular structure around the shoulder region and then the joints of the region can be understood. First notice the bony landmarks on the posterior aspect of the scapula (Fig. 1.28).

Seen from behind, it will immediately be obvious that the scapula is divided into upper and lower parts by a bony spine. This is the **scapular spine**, and it ends laterally as the **acromion**. The section of the scapula above this spine is the **supraspinous fossa** and the part below is the **infraspinous fossa**. The upper border of the scapula can now clearly be seen with its **scapular notch**. In fact this notch is converted into a foramen by a **suprascapular ligament**.

The two fossae on the back of the scapula communicate with each other deep to the lateral end of the spine by means of a **spinoglenoid notch**. Viewed from the back, three muscles can be seen immediately associated with the supraspinous and infraspinous fossae. These are the **supraspinatus** on the one hand and the **infraspinatus** and **teres minor** on the other (Fig. 1.29).

The supraspinatus arises from the supraspinous fossa and passes laterally beneath the overhanging acromion. Its tendon is inserted into the top of the greater tubercle of the humerus. Some of its fibres fuse with the capsule of the shoulder joint. Clinically the supraspinatus is an important muscle since rupture of its tendon may occur with injury. Also its tendon seems to be prone to calcific degeneration. Its relationships to the shoulder joint capsule on its undersurface and to the subacromial bursa on its upper surface (Fig. 1.30) are described in more detail with the account of the shoulder joint (see p. 19). A neurovascular bundle reaches the supraspinatus through the region of the scapular notch. The nerve is the **suprascapular nerve** from the brachial plexus in the neck. The arterial supply comes from a branch of the subclavian artery. The action of the muscle is to *abduct* the arm from the side of the body. It is the important muscle for *initiation* of this movement. With all the other muscles that surround the joint, it also adds to the stability of the shoulder joint.

The infraspinatus arises from the infraspinous fossa

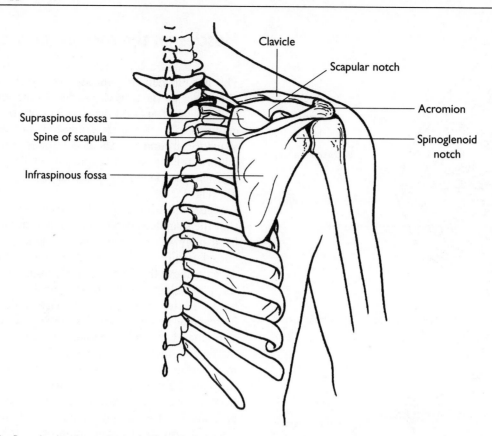

Figure 1.28 Bony landmarks on the back of the scapula.

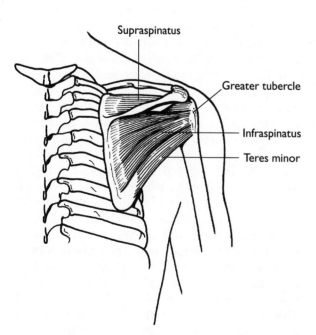

Figure 1.29 Muscles that arise from the back of the scapula.

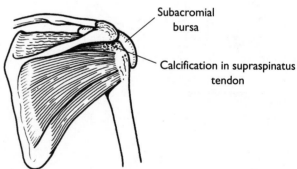

Figure 1.30 The subacromial bursa and supraspinatus tendon.

and is also inserted into the greater tubercle of the humerus. Some of its fibres blend with the shoulder joint capsule. It corresponds in position to the subscapularis on the front of the scapula. The muscle is supplied by the same neurovascular bundle that supplies the supraspinatus. This reaches the muscle by passing through the spinoglenoid notch. The infraspinatus is a *lateral rotator* of the arm (the opposite action to the subscapularis). It also adds to the stability of the joint.

The teres minor is a small muscle lying along the lower edge of the infraspinatus (Fig. 1.29). Its insertion and action are the same as those of the infraspinatus. It is, however, supplied with the nerve that supplies the deltoid, i.e. the axillary nerve. This is a good time to recall this nerve. It was last seen as a branch of the posterior cord of the brachial plexus. It left the axilla by squeezing between the subscapularis and teres major. It can now be seen more clearly from behind (Fig. 1.31).

From behind, three other muscles may be studied briefly. They suspend the scapula from the vertebral column and can rotate it on the chest wall. They are the **levator scapulae** and **rhomboid muscles** and the **trapezius** (Fig. 1.32). The levator scapulae and rhomboids arise from the vertebral column and insert into the medial edge of the scapula. They are supplied by the dorsal scapular nerve, a branch of the brachial plexus in the neck. They can draw the scapula towards the midline and also rotate the bone so that the glenoid cavity points downwards (Fig. 1.33). The tapezius arises from a long linear origin, taking in the back of the skull, the **ligamentum nuchae**, and the cervical and thoracic spines and their supraspinous ligaments (Fig. 1.32).

The upper fibres of the trapezius muscle descend over the shoulder to be inserted into the lateral third of the clavicle. The lower fibres pass to the acromion

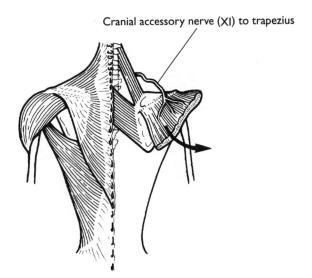

Figure 1.32 Trapezius retracted to reveal the cranial accessory nerve (XI) supplying it.

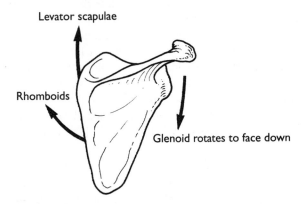

Figure 1.33 Muscles that rotate the glenoid cavity downwards.

and spine of the scapula. (This insertion is similar in extent to the origin of the deltoid.) The upper and lower parts of the trapezius act together to rotate the scapula so that the glenoid faces upwards (Fig. 1.34). The upper fibres acting alone elevate the whole of the scapula, and the middle fibres acting alone brace the shoulder backwards. The muscle is supplied by the spinal accessory nerve (part of the XI cranial nerve) in the neck.

The joints of the shoulder region

To appreciate the great mobility of the shoulder region three joints need to be studied. These are the

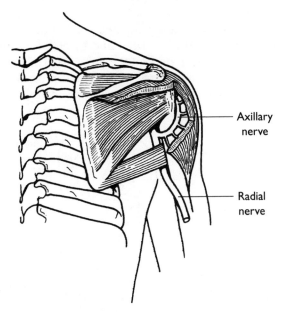

Figure 1.31 The deltoid muscle cut to reveal the axillary nerve with the radial nerve emerging beneath teres major.

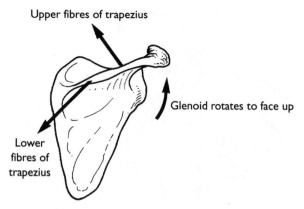

Figure 1.34 Muscles that rotate the glenoid cavity to face upwards.

sternoclavicular, the **acromioclavicular** and the **shoulder** joints (Fig. 1.35).

The sternoclavicular joint is a synovial joint which acts like a ball and socket. The ball is the medial end of the clavicle and the socket is formed by the strong manubrium and upper border of the first rib. These latter two structures are united by an immobile primary cartilaginous joint. The capsule of the joint is strong. The synovial cavity is usually divided by an intra-articular disc. The clavicle moves like a see-saw. When the shoulder is raised, the medial end of the clavicle is depressed; when the shoulder is braced backwards, the medial end projects forwards, and so on. The axis of this see-saw motion takes place through a strong ligament which binds the clavicle to the first rib. Circumduction at the sternoclavicular joint combines all these movements. Displacement of the joint is resisted by the strong ligaments and capsule and by the presence of the articular disc that divides the joint cavity into two. This disc is attached to the clavicle above and to the first rib below; it therefore prevents extreme upward displacement of the medial end of the clavicle. The sternoclavicular joint is the only articulation between the pectoral girdle and the trunk. The scapula articulates with the lateral end of the clavicle at the acromioclavicular joint. The stress of supporting the weight of the upper limb and its girdle, however, is taken by strong ligaments that bind the coracoid process to the clavicle. These are the **coracoclavicular ligaments** (Fig. 1.35). The scapula receives additional support from muscles such as the levator scapulae and trapezius which suspend it from the head, neck and trunk.

The acromioclavicular joint is a synovial joint which allows only a little gliding movement between its surfaces. The shoulder joint, however, is a synovial joint of the ball and socket variety. The bones involved are the head of the humerus and the glenoid cavity of the scapula. The head of the humerus is spherical but is limited at its periphery by a thick **'anatomical' neck**. If the bone is fractured during injury, it does not break across this neck but more usually across the thinner proximal shaft of the bone. This region is below the head and tubercles and is named the **'surgical' neck** of the humerus. The head of the humerus is covered with articular cartilage (Fig. 1.36). The glenoid cavity is pear-shaped and

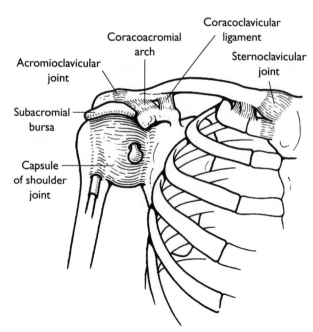

Figure 1.35 The three synovial joints of the shoulder region.

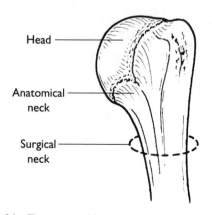

Figure 1.36 The proximal humerus.

slightly concave (Fig. 1.37) and at first sight it appears to be far too small and shallow to accept the head of the humerus. Its articular surface, however, is deepened slightly by a rim of fibrous tissue called the **labrum glenoidale**. The **capsule** of the joint is attached to both bones around their articular margins, i.e. to the labrum of the scapula and around the anatomical neck of the humerus. As the capsule bridges over the intertubercular groove, it is thickened to form the so-called **transverse ligament**. Inferiorly it is also worth noting that the capsule is in fact attached well below the anatomical neck.

The capsule has several holes through which synovial membrane can protrude (Fig. 1.35). In front, the **subscapular bursa** protrudes through a hole. A similar bursa is sometimes found beneath the infraspinatus at the back of the capsule. Synovial membrane also appears beneath the bridge formed by the transverse ligament. Here it covers a tendon which arises from the scapula, above the glenoid, and passes along the intertubercular groove into the upper arm. The tendon is that of the long head of the biceps muscle.

Certain ligaments help to strengthen the capsule. In places these are simply thickenings of the capsule itself. The **coracohumeral ligament** is a band of fibrous tissue which passes from the coracoid process to the greater tubercle. This ligament prevents excessive external rotation at the shoulder. Above the joint is a strong fibrous bridge. This is the **coracoacromial ligament**. With the coracoid process and the acromion it forms a strong arch above the joint, so preventing any upward displacement of the joint. The long head of biceps can also be thought of as an accessory 'ligament', since it passes over the humeral head, inside the joint, to the intertubercular groove. This part of its course is therefore intracapsular. By its position it also aids in stabilizing the joint.

Synovial membrane lines the inside of the capsule and all other intracapsular surfaces *except* those covered with articular cartilage. This means that within the shoulder joint, quite apart from the inner aspect of the capsule, it also covers the long head of the biceps tendon. Synovial membrane is also involved in the formation of the subscapular bursa. The subacromial bursa can also be noted at this stage. This bursa does *not* communicate with the joint synovia. It is a separate 'bag' of synovial membrane (Fig. 1.38). It covers the upper part of the joint capsule and the supraspinatus tendon which has fused with the capsule on its way to the greater tubercle. It separates this moving surface from the coracoacromial arch and deltoid muscles above.

The relations of the shoulder joint need to be studied carefully since they have a bearing on the surgical exposure of the joint and on its function. On all aspects, except for a small area below, the capsule is surrounded by muscles and their tendons. The tendons of these muscles all fuse with the capsule so forming a strong sleeve around the joint, which has been

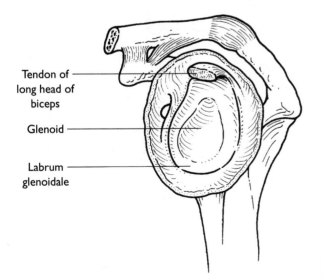

Figure 1.37 The glenoid cavity and labrum glenoidale.

Tendon of long head of biceps

Glenoid

Labrum glenoidale

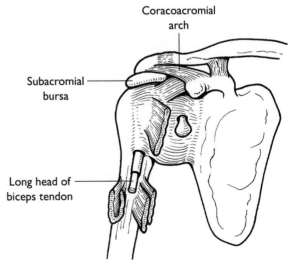

Coracoacromial arch

Subacromial bursa

Long head of biceps tendon

Figure 1.38 The subacromial bursa and long head of the biceps tendon surrounded by synovial membrane as it emerges from the joint capsule.

called the **rotator cuff** (Fig. 1.39). Above is the supraspinatus; behind is the infraspinatus (and teres minor). In front is the subscapularis.

Below, the capsule is unsupported and it falls as a fold between the lower borders of subscapularis and infraspinatus. If the shoulder joint is dislocated it usually does so through this weak inferior aspect, the head of the humerus being forced down into this part of the capsule. In this way it can injure the axillary nerve as it passes from the axilla between the subscapularis and teres major below.

In no other joint in the body is movement so free as in the shoulder joint. The freedom of movement results from the large rounded area of the head of the humerus in comparison with the small, shallow glenoid, and also the lax capsule surrounding the joint. Because of this freedom, the joint must be protected from dislocations during movements. Several things contribute to this. The most important stabilizing factor is the rotator cuff tendons. These muscles have a low mechanical advantage for movement of the shoulder; their prime function is to hold the head of the humerus in the glenoid cavity during movements of the arm. The overhanging coracoacromial arch also protects the upper part of the joint. Atmospheric pressure is said also to keep the joint surfaces together, but this can have little effect in preventing dislocations, since any dislocating force is a sliding force between the head and the glenoid rather than the joint surfaces simply falling apart.

Many types of movement occur at the shoulder joint. Flexion is a forward movement of the arm in the sagittal plane, extension being the opposite movement. In abduction the arm is lifted away from the body (Fig. 1.40) and in adduction the arm is brought back to the side of the body. A combination of all of these produces the movement of circumduction. This should not be confused with rotation at the joint. Rotation means that the humerus rotates in its long axis. Flexion is produced by the anterior fibres of the deltoid, aided by some fibres of pectoralis major. Extension on the other hand is produced by the posterior fibres of the deltoid, aided by some fibres of the latissimus dorsi. Abduction needs special study. Initially the supraspinatus abducts the arm, but then the strong deltoid takes over. If the supraspinatus is paralysed or torn, patients cannot initiate abduction. They soon learn a trick movement and swing the arm passively from the side to get up the initial momentum. When the shoulder joint is abducted to almost 90° the articular surface of the head is 'used up'. The head has to be rotated laterally to bring in more available articular surface. (The mechanism of abduction at the shoulder joint is shown in Fig. 1.40.) Adduction is produced by the pectoralis major and latissimus dorsi. Rotation of the humerus is achieved by the short scapular muscles, the subscapularis, teres major and infraspinatus.

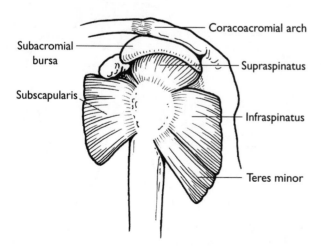

Figure 1.39 The muscles of the rotator cuff.

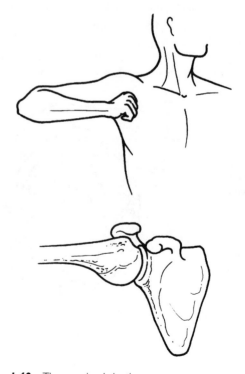

Figure 1.40 The arm in abduction.

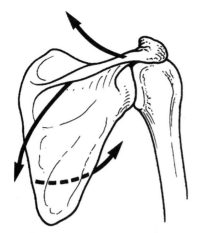

Figure 1.41 Rotation of the scapula during abduction at the shoulder joint.

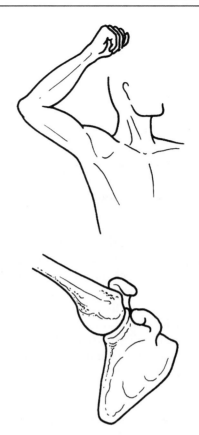

Figure 1.42 Depression of the clavicle and rotation of the scapula accompanying abduction of the humerus at the shoulder joint.

The essential point to understand when analysing movements of the shoulder region is that none of the three joints moves separately. Movement in one is always accompanied by movement in the other two. For example, during abduction there is not only movement in the shoulder joint itself but also rotation of the scapula (Fig. 1.41). This is produced by the trapezius and serratus anterior. These muscles rotate the scapula so that the glenoid points upwards (Fig. 1.42). With this elevation of the shoulder there is passive depression of the medial end of the clavicle at the sternoclavicular joint. You can confirm this while abducting your own arm. Feel the inferior angle of the scapula with the other hand. At a certain point during abduction you will feel the scapula begin its rotation. Now abduct the arm once again, and this time feel the medial end of the clavicle. During the abduction the see-saw effect will cause it to be depressed.

Applied anatomy of the pectoral region

The shoulder region is often injured and frequently patients present with fractures of the bones or dislocations of the joints. The breast is often the seat of carcinoma, and so you will have to examine this structure frequently. Abscesses and other simple lumps in the breast also have to be differentiated. Remember again that no examination of the breast is complete without an examination of the axilla. Palpation of axillary nodes that may be involved with carcinoma of the breast is of vital importance.

Injuries to the bones and joints of the shoulder region

There are two shoulders on every patient! If one is injured it is always good policy to examine the other for comparison. The clavicle is a bone that frequently fractures, especially amongst those who play sports. The fracture is usually medial to the coracoclavicular ligament. The pectoral girdle tends to fall with the outer third of the clavicle. The bone is put back into place simply by bracing the shoulders back and holding them there with a bandage. Luckily this type of fracture unites readily.

The humerus is often fractured across its surgical

neck. This is a fairly common type of fracture but it usually heals well. Dislocations may occur at the shoulder joint. Usually, the head of the humerus leaves the glenoid cavity travelling inferiorly, which is potentially injurious to the axillary nerve. The head of the humerus is usually drawn medially below and in front of the glenoid fossa by the powerful adductor muscles, so that the most prominent lateral bony landmark of the shoulder is now the acromion. Spasm in the subscapularis causes medial rotation of the humerus so that the elbow lies away from the body wall and the wrist is held against the body by the other hand. One method of reducing a dislocated shoulder is first to rotate the forearm outwards with the elbow flexed (which stretches the subscapularis) and then to bring the elbow medially across the trunk (which levers the head of the humerus laterally so that it slips back into the glenoid fossa). As soon as the shoulder is reduced, the sensory nerve supply to the area of skin overlying the deltoid tuberosity and the function of the deltoid muscle must be tested. If the skin is sensitive and the deltoid contracts, the axillary nerve is intact.

The supraspinatus tendon is sometimes injured during falls, and is torn near its insertion. The tendon then has to be repaired surgically. The supraspinatus tendon is also prone to degenerative changes. The degenerated parts become calcified and this causes pain when abduction is attempted and can also set up inflammation within the subacromial bursa.

Injury to the brachial plexus

The main causes of injury to the brachial plexus are cervical rib, birth injury and road traffic accidents. A great force hitting the shoulder may pull nerve roots away from the spinal cord in the neck. During our study of the vertebral column you will note that an extra 'cervical rib' can cause pressure on the 1st thoracic contribution to the brachial plexus as well as to the vessels travelling through the thoracic outlet to and from the upper limb. If undue traction is applied to the head and neck of a baby during delivery, injury to the brachial plexus may occur. The common type of injury is called the Erb–Duchenne syndrome. The injury commonly involves the upper trunk of the plexus (C5 and C6). The suprascapular branch is also involved since it arises from the plexus at this point, and the infant has a deformity of the upper limb as a result of the injury. Occasionally it is the middle trunk (C7) that is injured. This produces paralysis of most of the muscles supplied by the radial nerve. If the lower trunk is injured (C8, T1) one of the main effects is paralysis of the small muscles of the hand (Klumpke syndrome).

chapter 2

The Upper Arm and Elbow Joint

The bone of the upper arm is the humerus and we need to study the **shaft of the humerus** along with its distal end. On the front of the shaft there are no important features. However, on the posterior aspect of the bone there is an oblique marking that is important to note. It is called the **radial groove**, and will be referred to later. In the elbow region, there are several interesting bony features. Seen from the front, the lateral and medial borders of the humerus become sharp margins and then project as **lateral** and **medial epicondyles** (Fig. 2.1). The medial epicondyle is always the more prominent of the two.

The lower end of the humerus presents two cartilage-covered surfaces. On the lateral side there is the **capitulum**, a rounded eminence that articulates with the head of the forearm bone, called the **radius**. On the medial side there is a larger, pulley-shaped process called the **trochlea**. This articulates with the **ulna**, the other forearm bone. The humerus is excavated above the capitulum and trochlea to form two fossae. The trochlea can be seen in a posterior view of the bones (Fig. 2.2). The capitulum, however, does not extend on to this surface of the humerus and is seen only from the front. Above the trochlea, the posterior surface of the humerus is also excavated to form a fossa.

The two forearm bones are the radius and ulna. The upper end of the **radius** is expanded into a cylindrical, cartilage-covered **head**. The constricted part below the head is called the **neck** of the radius. Just below the neck on the medial aspect is a prominent **radial tuberosity**. The upper end of the **ulna** clasps the trochlea. This can be best appreciated by looking at a side view of the bones (Fig. 2.3). The process projecting around the posterior aspect of the trochlea is called the **olecranon**. The anterior projection in front

of the trochlea of the ulna is called the **coronoid process**. Just distal to the coronoid process there is a tuberosity on the ulna.

The **capitulum** articulates with the upper surface of the radial head. The periphery of the radial head fits into a **radial notch** at the side of the ulna. Both of these surfaces are also covered with articular cartilage. The trochlea articulates with the **trochlear notch** of the ulna. Having defined the limits of the trochlear fossa as the coronoid process in front and the olecra-

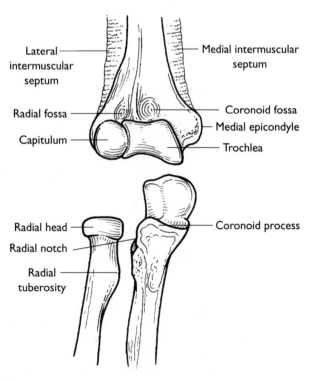

Figure 2.1 Anterior view of the bones at the elbow.

Lateral intermuscular septum

Medial intermuscular septum

Radial fossa

Coronoid fossa

Capitulum

Medial epicondyle

Trochlea

Radial head

Coronoid process

Radial notch

Radial tuberosity

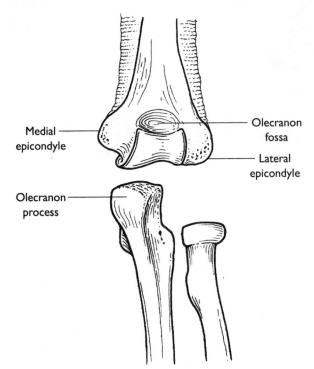

Medial epicondyle

Olecranon fossa

Lateral epicondyle

Olecranon process

Figure 2.2   Posterior view of the bones at the elbow.

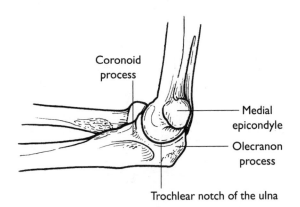

Coronoid process

Medial epicondyle

Olecranon process

Trochlear notch of the ulna

Figure 2.3   Medial side of the elbow joint.

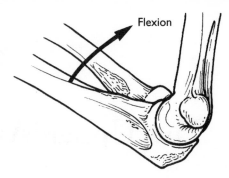

Flexion

Figure 2.4   Flexion of the forearm at the elbow joint brings the coronoid process and head of the radius into close proximity with the radial and coronoid fossae.

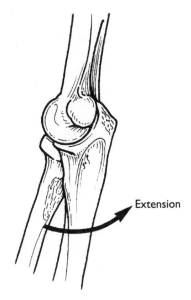

Extension

Figure 2.5   Extension of the forearm at the elbow joint brings the olecranon into close proximity with the olecranon fossa of the humerus.

non behind, the reasons for the excavations in the humerus may now be easily understood (Fig. 2.4). With flexion of the elbow, the coronoid process abuts on to the humerus. The so-called **coronoid fossa** therefore accepts this process in extreme flexion. Similarly, with full extension at the elbow (Fig. 2.5) the olecranon fits into the **olecranon fossa**. On the lateral side, the head of the radius fits into the **radial fossa** when the elbow is flexed. In extension, however, it

does not reach as far back as the olecranon and so there is no radial fossa on the posterior aspect of the humerus.

Identify the bony landmarks on radiographs of the elbow (Figs 2.6 and 2.7). The upper arm consists of muscles that are responsible for flexing and extending the elbow joint. The **flexor muscles** are found at the front of the humerus and the **extensor muscles** at the back. On either side of the humerus there is a condensation of connective tissue between these two sets of muscles. This gives the impression of two septa which stretch from the margins of the humerus to the sleeve of deep fascia surrounding the arm (Fig. 2.8). They are called the **medial** and **lateral intermuscular septa**.

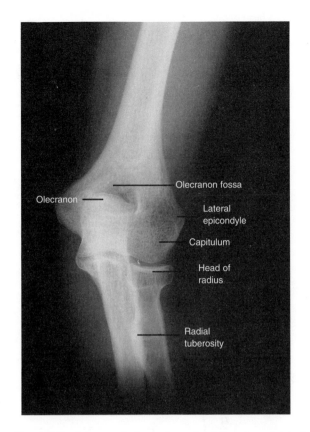

Figure 2.6 Anteroposterior radiograph of the elbow joint. A few key landmarks are labelled.

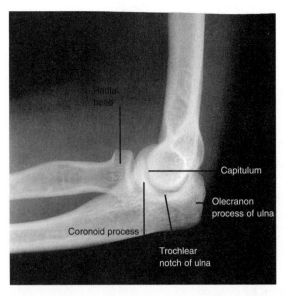

Figure 2.7 Lateral radiograph of the elbow joint. Key landmarks are labelled.

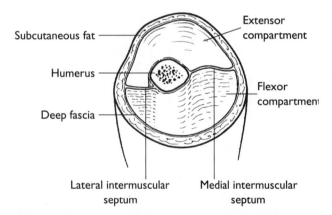

Figure 2.8 The flexor and extensor compartments of the upper arm.

For convenience, therefore, the upper arm may be thought of as having two compartments: the anterior compartment containing the flexor musculature and the posterior with the extensor muscles.

The terminal branches of the brachial plexus weave through these two compartments. The lateral and medial cords supply flexor aspects of the upper limb, and the posterior cord innervates extensor parts. In the case of the upper arm it is a branch of the lateral cord that supplies the flexor musculature. The other terminal branches of the lateral and medial cords are merely passing through the upper arm to reach flexor parts of the forearm and hand. The extensor musculature of the upper arm is supplied by the radial nerve, which is the only remaining branch of the posterior cord once it has left the axilla.

Musculature of the anterior compartment

Three muscles are found on the front of the humerus in the upper arm. They are the **coracobrachialis**, the **biceps brachii** and the **brachialis** muscles. The **coracobrachialis** is a small insignificant muscle in humans. It arises from the coracoid process and is inserted halfway down the shaft of the humerus (Fig. 2.9). It is a weak adductor of the shoulder joint. Powerful adduction at the shoulder has been taken over by the pectoralis major and latissimus dorsi muscles.

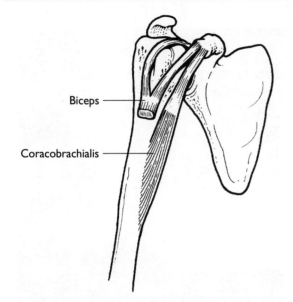

Figure 2.9 The tendons of origin of biceps and coracobrachialis.

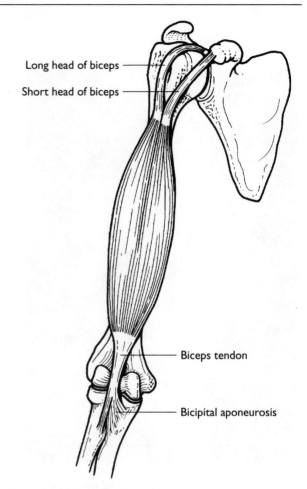

Figure 2.10 The biceps muscle.

The **biceps** and **brachialis** are much more important muscles to study. They are both flexors of the elbow joint. The **biceps** arises by two heads (Figs 2.9 and 2.10). The long head arises from the **supraglenoid tubercle** of the scapula just above the apex of the glenoid cavity. It passes over the upper end of the humerus inside the capsule of the shoulder joint. It leaves the interior of the joint by passing along the intertubercular groove underneath the transverse ligament. While in the shoulder joint it is covered by synovial membrane. The **short** head arises from the coracoid process in common with the coracobrachialis. Both heads unite in the upper arm and give rise to a powerful muscle which is easily seen in the living limb. The muscle is inserted into *both* forearm bones. Its main insertion is into the radial tuberosity by means of a strong tendon. This can easily be palpated in the living limb. From the medial border of this tendon a thin aponeurosis spreads into the deep fascia and blends with the periosteum on the ulna. This is the insertion into the ulna.

Place your forearm flat on the table with the palm facing upwards. In this position the radius and ulna lie side by side and more or less parallel to each other. Keep the elbow flexed to a right angle. Ask someone to hold the hand against the table in this position and then try to raise the forearm into full flexion against this resistance. With your other hand you will be able to feel the taught biceps tendon and the edge of the

bicipital aponeurosis. Acting in this way the biceps flexes the elbow by pulling on both forearm bones. The biceps muscle, however, has a further action. With the elbow at right angles and the forearm resting on the table, turn your hand over so that the palm now is facing down on to the table. In this position the radius and ulna no longer lie parallel but are crossed. The biceps can now pull on the radius by means of its tendon and uncross the bones, once more bringing the palm to face upwards. This movement of crossed forearm bones to uncrossed is called **supination**. It is the movement that is used in screwing a screw into a piece of wood. With the elbow flexed, go though the motions of putting in a screw and at the same time feel the biceps muscle. Each time the screw is 'tightened' you will feel the muscle contract. Last describes these two functions of the biceps graphically when he writes: 'the muscle puts *in* the cork screw (supination) and then pulls *out* the cork (flexion)' (Last RJ (1972) *Anatomy Regional and Applied*, 5th edn. Churchill Livingstone). Note, however, that this analogy applies to you only if you are right handed! The long head of the biceps also helps to keep the head of the humerus in the glenoid cavity.

The **brachialis** is a much simpler muscle to study. It arises from the distal half of the shaft of the humerus and intermuscular septa (Figs 2.11 and 2.12). The fibres are inserted into the coronoid process of the ulna. The muscle is therefore a simple *flexor* of the elbow joint.

Neurovascular structures in the anterior compartment

The vessels and nerves descending from the axilla weave their way between the three muscles of the upper arm. At the lower extremity of the axilla the axillary artery is surrounded by the cords of the brachial plexus. The lateral cord gives off the musculocutaneous branch and then continues on as the median nerve. The medial cord continues as the ulnar nerve (Fig. 2.13). Behind the artery lies the radial nerve, the continuation of the posterior cord. On the medial side of the artery is the axillary vein. All

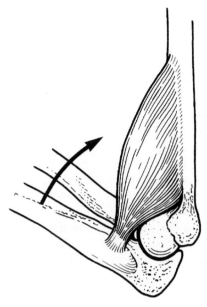

Figure 2.12 Brachialis acts to flex the elbow.

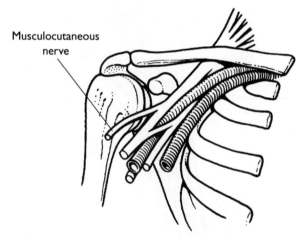

Musculocutaneous nerve

Figure 2.13 The origin of the musculocutaneous nerve from the lateral cord of the brachial plexus.

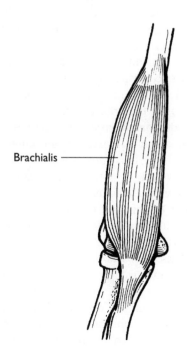

Brachialis —

Figure 2.11 The brachialis muscle.

three muscles of the anterior compartment are supplied by the **musculocutaneous nerve**. The musculocutaneous nerve was noted earlier as it entered the combined biceps and coracobrachialis muscles. It supplies both of these muscles and then continues under cover of the biceps to reach the brachialis muscle. After supplying this muscle, only sensory fibres remain, and these may be found as a lateral cutaneous nerve emerging to the surface from beneath the lower part of the lateral border of the biceps. It supplies skin of the forearm.

The other two nerves that arise from the lateral and medial cords are the ulnar nerve and the median nerve. Both the ulnar and median nerves are simple nerves of passage in the upper arm. They descend to supply muscles and skin in the flexor parts of the forearm and hand. They therefore have no branches in the upper arm. The **ulnar nerve**, during its passage through the upper arm, 'wanders' for a short distance into the posterior compartment. By doing this it is able to negotiate the elbow region. Below the elbow it naturally returns to the flexor aspect of the forearm. It therefore leaves the medial side of the axillary artery and pierces the medial intermuscular septum (Fig. 2.14). It descends behind the septum and behind the medial epicondyle of the humerus. It can be palpated here in the arm as a thick cord at the back of the medial epicondyle. It then re-enters the flexor compartment below the elbow. The **median nerve** stays in the flexor compartment during its descent through the upper arm. It simply passes down to the front of the elbow, overlapped and covered by the biceps. In the lower part of the upper arm it rests on the brachialis muscle. In its descent, the nerve is accompanied by the artery of the arm, which is now renamed the **brachial artery** (Fig. 2.14). The artery can be palpated in the living upper arm at the medial side of the biceps if this muscle is gently pushed aside. The median nerve and brachial artery thus form a neurovascular bundle. They cross one another as they pass through the upper arm, sometimes the nerve crossing in front of the artery and sometimes behind. However, when they reach the front of the elbow the median nerve always lies to the medial side of the brachial artery.

The brachial artery is accompanied by **venae comitantes**. These also receive superficial venous tributaries so that, by the time the axilla is reached, a single axillary vein is formed at the medial side of the artery. The brachial artery gives muscular branches in the upper arm and supplies the humerus through a nutrient artery. For the most part its branches follow the main nerves and many end by anastomosing around the sides of the elbow with forearm branches. Thus a vascular network is formed around the elbow joint. Above, it also gives branches that anastomose with the circumflex vessels. The names of these branches need not be remembered. The brachial artery does give one large consistent branch called the **profunda brachii**. This is the branch that accompanies the radial nerve into the posterior compartment of the upper arm. The **radial nerve** passes into the posterior compartment to supply the extensor musculature of the upper arm (Fig. 2.15). After supplying this musculature, however, it re-enters the anterior compartment by piercing the lateral intermuscular septum (Fig. 2.14). It thus passes to the forearm in front of the elbow. But here it divides into muscular and cutaneous branches, both of which pass once again into the extensor aspects of the forearm and hand.

The two cutaneous branches of the medial cord travel towards the skin in the upper arm, the **medial cutaneous nerve of the arm** supplying skin in the upper arm and the **medial cutaneous nerve of the forearm** supplying skin in the more distal parts of the limb.

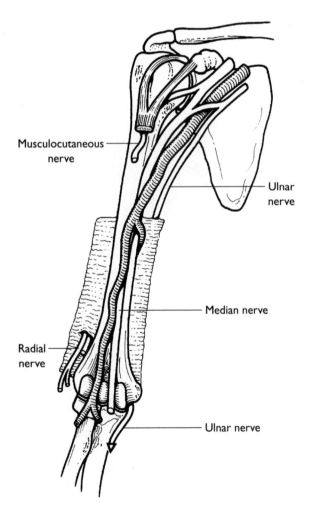

Musculocutaneous nerve

Ulnar nerve

Median nerve

Radial nerve

Ulnar nerve

Figure 2.14 The ulnar and median nerves in the upper arm.

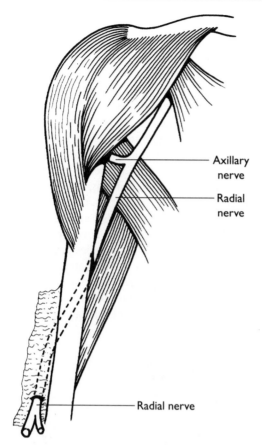

Figure 2.15 The radial nerve passing behind the humerus.

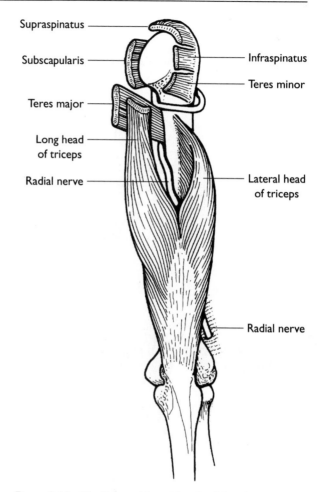

Figure 2.16 The long and lateral heads of the triceps muscle.

Musculature of the posterior compartment

There is but one muscle in the posterior compartment of the upper arm: it is the extensor of the elbow joint called the **triceps** muscle. As its name suggests, it arises by means of three heads (Fig. 2.16). The long head arises from the scapula and the other two from the back of the humerus.

The triceps muscle is formed in two strata. The superficial stratum consists of the **long** and **lateral heads** of the muscle. The long head arises from **infraglenoid tubercle** of the scapula just below the glenoid cavity. The lateral head has a linear origin from the back of the humerus just above the radial groove. These two heads unite to form a bulky muscle mass at the back of the upper arm. In order to see the third head, the conjoined long and lateral heads must be split because the third head arises deep to the superficial muscular stratum (Fig. 2.17). It should therefore

be called the 'deep' head but unfortunately it is poorly named. It is actually called the **medial head** of the triceps. It arises from the back of the humerus and intermuscular septa below the level of the radial groove. It therefore has a similar origin on the back of the humerus to the brachialis on the front. The fibres of all three heads unite to form a strong tendon which is inserted into the olecranon. A small bursa separates the tendon from the capsule of the elbow joint. The triceps muscle is the extensor of the elbow joint. Its long head, however, gives support to the shoulder joint when the arm is abducted (Fig. 2.18). The muscle, being an extensor, is supplied by the posterior cord of the brachial plexus, that is by the **radial nerve**.

At this point it is worth mentioning a small muscle called the **anconeus**, which should really be thought of as part of the triceps muscle. It arises from the posterior aspect of the lateral epicondyle of the humerus and is partially blended with the triceps here. It inserts into the lateral side of the olecranon and proximal portion of the posterior surface of the ulna. The anconeus abducts the ulna during pronation of the forearm. It also acts with the triceps to extend the elbow joint. During flexion of the elbow the anconeus is active as a stabilizer of the elbow joint. Naturally, it is supplied by the radial nerve.

The **radial nerve** leaves the posterior aspect of the axillary artery and passes to the back of the humerus (Fig. 2.15). It is accompanied by the profunda brachii artery. On the back of the humerus it lies under a muscular roof made up of the long and lateral heads of the triceps (Fig. 2.16). Under cover of these it takes an oblique course along the radial groove. It is, however, usually separated from the bone by a few fibres of the deep head of triceps. It supplies branches to all three heads of the triceps. On the lateral side of the humerus it pierces the lateral intermuscular septum, as already noted. In the anterior part of the arm it divides into cutaneous and muscular branches (Figs 2.14 and 2.19).

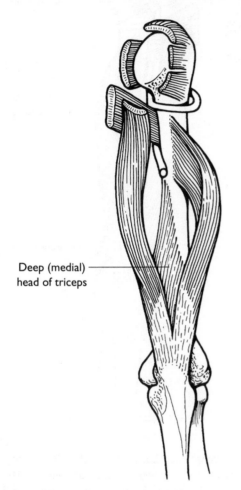

Deep (medial) head of triceps

Figure 2.17   The medial head of the triceps muscle exposed beneath the long and lateral heads.

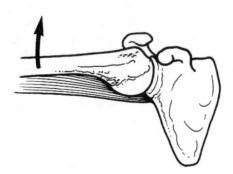

Figure 2.18   The long head of triceps supports the shoulder joint when the arm is abducted.

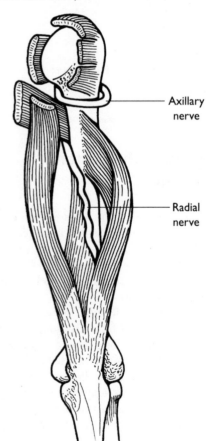

Axillary nerve

Radial nerve

Figure 2.19   The radial nerve in the radial groove on the posterior aspect of the humerus.

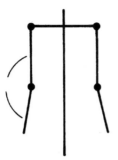

Figure 2.20 The carrying angle between the upper arm and forearm.

The elbow joint

The elbow joint is a synovial joint of the hinge variety. The articulation takes place between the lower end of the humerus and the upper ends of the radius and ulna. The articular surface of the humerus is divided into two parts. The trochlear is the pulley-shaped surface for articulation with the trochlear notch of the ulna, and it is the capitulum that articulates with the radial head (Fig. 2.1). The medial flange of the trochlea is lower than the lateral so that, when the ulna articulates with it, an angle is formed between the upper arm and forearm. The angle is called the 'carrying angle' since it is best seen when a weight is carried. The elbow fits into the waist, and the forearm is angulated away from the prominence of the hip (Fig. 2.20). The distal articular surface of the elbow joint is also separated into two parts. The upper surface of the radial head is covered with articular cartilage and this articulates with the capitulum of the humerus (Fig. 2.21). The upper grooved end of the

ulna, the trochlear notch, is the other part of this surface, and articulates with the trochlea. It is also covered with articular cartilage. The articulation between the side of the radial head and the radial notch of the ulna is *not* considered to be part of the elbow joint. However, note that this joint is held together by a strong band which passes as a loop around the head and neck of the radius from the anterior and posterior edges of the radial notch. The movements taking place in this joint are of course completely different to the simple hinge type of movement that occurs in the elbow joint proper. The fibrous loop around the radius is called the **annular ligament**.

The capsule and ligaments of the elbow joint

Since the elbow is a hinge joint it must be strong at the sides to prevent abnormal movements of the joint. But the anterior and posterior parts of the joint capsule are not so strong. The anterior fibres of the capsule pass from the epicondyles and upper margins of the coronoid and radial fossae above, to the coronoid process and annular ligament below. These fossae are therefore intracapsular (Fig. 2.22). Posteriorly, the capsule extends from the humerus, above the olecra-

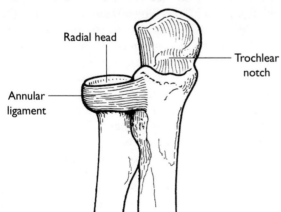

Figure 2.21 The annular ligament holds the head of the radius against the radial notch of the ulna.

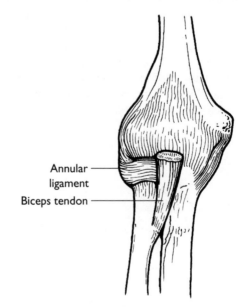

Figure 2.22 The capsule of the elbow joint seen from the front.

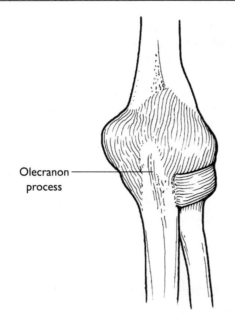

Olecranon process

Figure 2.23   The capsule of the elbow joint seen from behind.

non fossa, to the olecranon process below. The olecranon fossa is therefore also intracapsular (Fig. 2.23). A bursa separates the posterior capsule from the tendon of insertion of the triceps muscle.

On either side of the joint there are strong **collateral ligaments**. The **radial collateral ligament** is a strong band that passes from the lateral epicondyle above to the annular ligament below. The **ulnar collateral ligament** is made up from two bands that arise from the lateral epicondyle. The anterior band passes to the coronoid process and the fan-like posterior band to the olecranon (Fig. 2.24). Some fibres of the capsule run between the olecranon and coronoid processes forming an oblique band which effectively deepens the trochlear notch. The ulnar nerve, as it passes

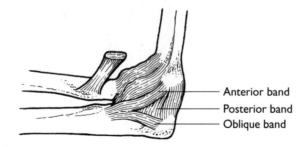

Anterior band
Posterior band
Oblique band

Figure 2.24   The three bands that make up the ulnar collateral ligament. The anterior band tightens in extension and the posterior band tightens in flexion. The oblique band deepens the trochlear notch.

around the medial epicondyle, lies on the ulnar collateral ligament. **Synovial membrane** lines the capsule and non-articular parts of the interior of the elbow joint. This means that folds of synovium actually cover the fossae. There are also fat pads between the synovial membrane and the capsule which bulge into the fossae when the bony prominences of the radius and ulna are withdrawn. Inferiorly, the synovial membrane is continuous with that of the joint between the radius and radial notch of the ulnar (the proximal radioulnar joint).

The movements that occur at the elbow joint are those of flexion and extension. If the anatomical position is assumed, flexion is a forward movement of the forearm and extension is a backward movement. Flexion is produced by the brachialis and biceps muscles. (These are assisted by several forearm muscles which arise from the epicondyles and pass into the forearm and hand.) Extension is produced by the triceps and anconeus muscles. (These are also assisted by several muscles arising from the lateral epicondyle and passing into the back of the forearm and hand.)

Applied anatomy of the upper arm and elbow joint

Fractures of the humerus are not uncommon. The pattern of the fracture and the fracture site depends on the type of injury and the age of the patient. Figure 2.25 shows three important types of fractures of the humerus. The bone can break across its 'surgical neck' (Fig. 2.25a). Travelling around this region is the axillary nerve and a vascular leash. Sometimes this type of fracture accompanies dislocation of the shoulder and only a radiograph will reveal the dual injury. The midshaft of the humerus may also be broken (Fig. 2.25b). In this type of injury the radial nerve may be injured as it passes along the radial groove at the back of the humerus. It has been estimated that this happens in about 8% of 'such fractures. It is important therefore to test for the integrity of the radial nerve in all patients who present with such a midshaft fracture of the humerus. If the radial nerve has been affected the patient will be unable to use the extensors of the wrist and fingers since the radial nerve supplies these muscles below the elbow. The patient presents with **wrist drop** and inability to

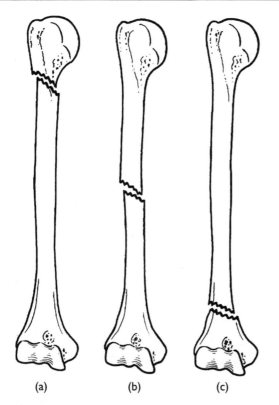

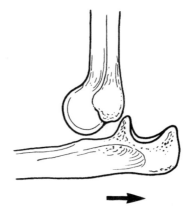

Figure 2.26 A dislocated elbow joint where the trochlear notch has slipped backwards relative to the shaft of the humerus.

(a)   (b)   (c)

Figure 2.25 (a) Fracture of the surgical neck of the humerus. (b) Midshaft fracture of the humerus. (c) Supracondylar fracture of the humerus.

extend the fingers actively. There will also be some sensory loss. The radial nerve gives a cutaneous branch to the lateral side of the arm and to the posterior surface of the forearm. These arise from the nerve as it is passing along the radial groove. Fracture of the shaft may occur above or below the level at which these cutaneous branches arise and so they may or may not be involved in the injury. However, the radial nerve gives a cutaneous branch to the radial side of the dorsum of the hand, and this arises in the forearm. If the radial nerve is interrupted by fracture of the humeral shaft there is therefore always a loss of sensation over the dorsum of the hand.

Motor and sensory losses following radial nerve interruption may result from other things besides fractures of the humeral shaft. This happened in the past following prolonged use of the old types of crutches. The nerve was compressed high in its course as it was leaving the axilla. In these cases the triceps could also loose its nerve supply. A similar situation sometimes follows the consumption of large volumes

of alcohol. On reaching his or her home, the subject then proceeds to fall sleep on a chair with an arm hanging over the sharp edge of the chair back. This type of injury is known in the trade as 'Saturday night paralysis'. The radial nerve may also be injured by bad placement of an arm on the operating table. Pressure on the nerve then brings about a radial nerve paralysis. Intramuscular injections, destined for the deltoid muscle, have sometimes been given into or around the radial nerve by the inexperienced.

The type of fracture depicted in Figure 2.25c may result from a fall. This is usually called a supracondylar fracture and occurs commonly in children. A lot of swelling occurs around the fracture site and, if the elbow is flexed to a right angle and held there during treatment, the pressure that builds up can cause compression of the brachial artery as it lies in front of the elbow. It is therefore important, after manipulation and immobilization in a sling, to examine such a child's pulse at regular intervals in order to recognize this serious complication. The median nerve is occasionally injured in this type of fracture in front of the elbow. An isolated fracture of the medial epicondyle can injure the ulnar nerve as it passes this region. The elbow joint is sometimes dislocated following an injury. Here the trochlear notch slips backwards (Fig. 2.26). Two clinical conditions concerning the olecranon may be noted. An enlarged bursa may appear beneath the skin following the oft-repeated trauma of resting the elbows on a table. The condition is called **olecranon bursitis**. The olecranon itself may be fractured transversely so that the triceps is then unable to extend the elbow.

The Forearm, Wrist, Hand and Digits

The forearm and wrist are concerned with spatial orientation of the hand so that the digits are able to perform complex and delicate movements in many positions relative to the rest of the body. You have only to watch the fingers and thumbs of, for example, a typist, watchmaker or pianist to appreciate how skillfully this can be done.

Bones, radiographs and joints of the forearm

The bones of the forearm are the **radius** and **ulna**. The **radius** lies on the lateral side of the forearm (assuming the forearm is supinated with the hand in the anatomical position). It is perhaps easier just to remember that the radius lies on the 'thumb' side of the forearm.

The head and neck of the radius have already been described. The head articulates with the radial notch on the ulna to form the **proximal radioulnar joint** (Fig. 3.1). The radius is held in place here against the ulna by a fibrous loop called the **annular ligament**. The lower edge of this ligament is attached very loosely to the neck of the radius. The lower part of this synovial joint is weak and a small ligament therefore extends between the lower margin of the radial notch and the neck of the radius. It is called the **quadrate ligament** (Fig. 3.2). The synovial membrane of the proximal radioulnar joint is an extension of the synovium of the elbow joint. The two cavities are therefore continuous.

Traced distally, the radius thickens whilst the ulna

becomes narrower (Fig. 3.3). The distal ends of the two bones may be felt as two bony prominences on either side of the wrist. These are called the **styloid processes** of the ulnar and radius. Notice on your

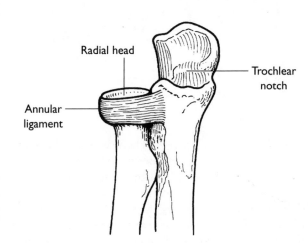

Figure 3.1 The proximal radioulnar joint between the head of the radius and the ulna.

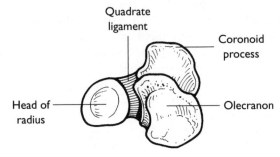

Figure 3.2 The quadrate ligament extends between the neck of the radius and the radial notch of the ulna.

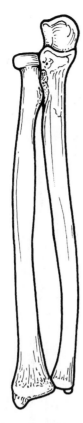

Figure 3.3 Distally, the radius thickens as the ulna narrows.

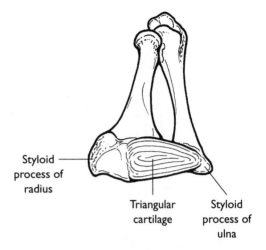

Figure 3.4 The triangular articular cartilage converges to a pointed apex on the styloid process of the ulna.

wrist that the radial styloid is lower than the ulnar styloid. This fact becomes important when examining a patient with a suspected fracture of the lower radius.

The distal end of the ulna, or head of the ulna, articulates with the **ulnar notch** of the radius at the **distal radioulnar joint**. This is another synovial joint. The joint has a very lax capsule but uniting the lower surface of the two bones is a **triangular cartilage** (Fig. 3.4). The triangular cartilage extends from a broad base on the lower end of the radius to a pointed apex on the ulnar styloid. The lower end of the radius together with the triangular cartilage make up the proximal articular surface of the wrist joint.

The forearm bones are able to twist around their long axis and so realign the hand and fingers distally. These twisting movements are called **supination** (for example when twisting in the direction of screwing in a cork screw with your right hand) and **pronation** (twisting the opposite way in the direction of unscrewing with your right hand). During these movements *the ulna remains stationary.* (This is not

absolutely true, but it is easier for you to understand things if you simply assume this for now.)

During supination and pronation the distal radius describes a cone of movement around the stationary ulna. For this to take place, rotation of the radial head must occur in the radial notch (i.e. at the proximal radioulnar joint). The annular ligament ensures that the radial head cannot drift away from its notch on the ulna. At the distal radioulnar joint the lower end of the radius swings around the stationary lower end of the ulna. The axis of movement is therefore through a line drawn from the middle of the head of the radius to the styloid process of the ulna (Fig. 3.5) where the apex of the triangular cartilage attaches.

Consider the forearm in the supinated position (Fig. 3.5). In this case, the thumb is pointing laterally and the two forearm bones are flat and parallel. (The radial tuberosity is clearly seen on a radiograph when the forearm is supinated.) To move into the pronated position, the radius must rotate at its head while its lower end swings around the ulna carrying the triangular articular disc and hand with it. The movement has described a 'cone', the apex being at the radial head and the base of the cone being circumscribed by the styloid of the radius. In the pronated position (Fig. 3.6) the thumb points medially and the two bones are crossed. (The radial tubercle is not easily seen on the radiograph when the forearm is pronated, since it has rotated around the back with the radial movement.)

A fibrous membrane exists between the two forearm bones and ties their shafts together (Fig. 3.7). It

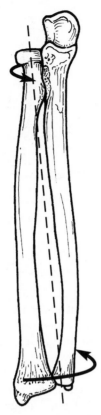

Figure 3.5 Supinated forearm bones lie flat. The arrows in the diagram illustrate that during pronation the distal radius describes a cone of movement around the stationary ulna.

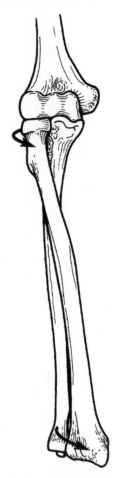

Figure 3.6 The forearm bones in the pronated position.

is called the **interosseous membrane**. Its fibres pass obliquely down from the radius to the ulna. During much of the movements of pronation and supination it is quite lax and therefore does not 'hold' the bones together in this sense. Its function is to provide increased area for the origin of forearm muscles. Thus, often, forearm muscles originate from the interosseous membrane as well as from the forearm bones.

So far we have studied the arm, elbow and forearm in the anatomical position (Fig. 3.8a). However, many people prefer to study the hand in the position shown in Figure 3.8b. They argue that this is the position of the hand during clinical examination. In truth, the hand may be studied in either orientation *provided* the forearm is also studied in the same orientation. Many of the tendons and nerves of the forearm pass straight into the wrist, hand and fingers so that it becomes confusing to think of the forearm in the anatomical position and the hand in another position as shown in Figure 3.8b. Here, we simply choose to continue to describe the forearm, wrist, hand and fingers in the anatomical position.

The bones of the wrist

The bones of the wrist are called the **carpal bones** and they are arranged in two rows (Fig. 3.9). The **proximal row** of carpal bones are the **scaphoid**, **lunate** and **triquetrum**. These bones are united by ligaments so that together they form a smooth, arched surface. The articulation between these bones and the lower end of the radius is called the **wrist joint**. The wrist joint is a synovial joint.

The proximal articular surface of the wrist joint is the concave lower end of the radius. This is extended medially as the triangular articular cartilage. The apex of the triangular cartilage is attached to the

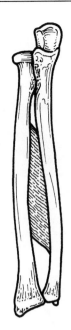

Figure 3.7 The interosseous membrane ties the shafts of the forearm bones together.

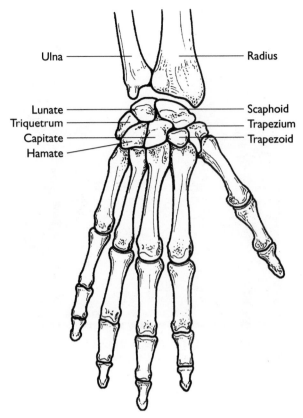

Figure 3.9 The carpal bones.

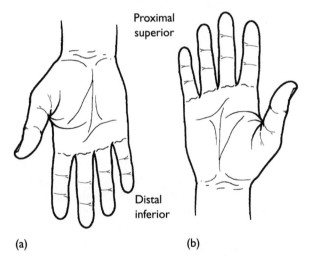

Figure 3.8 (a) The hand in the anatomical position; (b) the hand as often presented in clinical examination.

styloid process of the ulna (Fig. 3.4). The ulna, therefore, takes no part in the formation of the wrist joint proper. The distal articular surface of the wrist joint is made up of the scaphoid, lunate and triquetrum. In fact the triquetrum comes into contact with the articular cartilage only when the wrist is bent into adduction. Identify on a radiograph the bones that form the wrist joint (Fig. 3.10). Notice on the lateral film (Fig. 3.11) that the lower end of the radius is

obliquely placed, sloping palmwards a little. This is an important point to remember when 'setting' the lower end of the radius following a fracture.

A **fibrous capsule** surrounds the wrist joint and is thickened on either side as the **radial** and **ulnar collateral ligaments**. The **synovial membrane**, as always, lines the inside of the capsule. The wrist may be flexed, extended (Fig. 3.12), abducted and adducted (Fig. 3.13). A combination movement of these results in circumduction. However, rotation in the long axis of the forearm is *not* possible. A joint of this type, which allows all movements except rotation, is called a **condyloid** type of synovial joint.

During **adduction** the hand moves towards the body, but remember that the arm must be in the anatomical position, i.e. with the palm of the hand facing forwards. During this movement the proximal row of carpal bones slides so that the triquetrum comes into contact with the triangular articular cartilage. **Abduction** of the wrist is not as free as adduction since the scaphoid comes into contact with the radial styloid (Fig. 3.13).

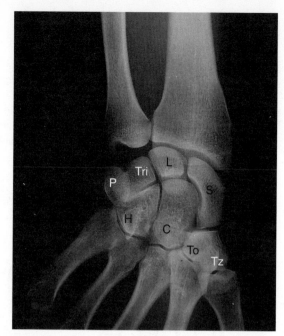

Figure 3.10 A radiograph of the wrist joint showing the carpal bones. S, scaphoid; L, lunate; Tri, triquetrum; P, pisiform; H, lies over the hook of the hamate; C, capitate; To, trapezoid; Tz, trapezium.

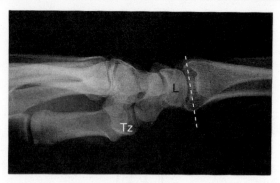

Figure 3.11 A lateral radiograph of the wrist joint illustrating the oblique orientation of the distal end of the radius as indicated by the dotted line. L, lunate; Tz, trapezium. The saddle-shaped nature of the joint between the trapezium and the thumb metacarpal is apparent.

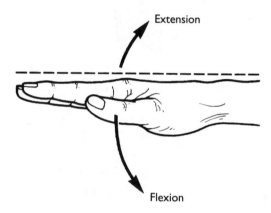

Figure 3.12 Flexion and extension at the wrist joint.

The distal row of carpal bones consists of four small bones called the **trapezium**, **trapezoid**, **capitate** and **hamate** (Fig. 3.9). Identify them on a radiograph of the wrist in Figure 3.10.

The trapezium and trapezoid are roughly cube-shaped; the capitate is larger and extends into the concavity of the proximal row. The hamate is characterized by having a bony hook on its palmar surface. The bones of the two rows of the carpus articulate with one another as a complex synovial joint. This joint is called the **midcarpal joint**. A fibrous capsule surrounds the joint, and certain ligaments join each bone to its neighbours (Fig. 3.14). The details of these ligaments need not be learned. Movement between

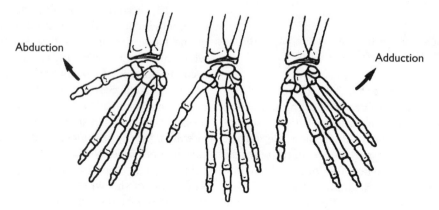

Figure 3.13 Abduction and adduction at the wrist joint.

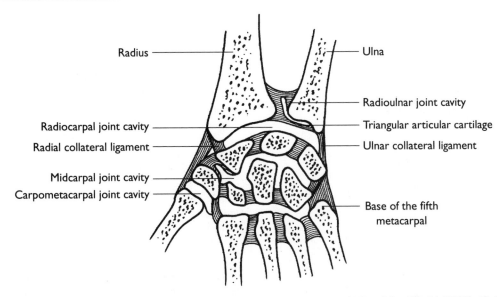

Figure 3.14 The ligaments and joint capsules of the wrist, carpal and carpometacarpal joints (after Ellis, H. (1983) *Clinical Anatomy*, 7th edn. Oxford: Blackwell).

the carpal bones is of a gliding nature. These gliding movements increase the flexibility of the wrist during movement. There is gliding movement between the two rows of carpal bones themselves. Five bony struts articulate with the distal row of carpal bones. These are the five **metacarpals** and they form the bony framework of the palm of the hand. The articulations between the metacarpals and the carpal bones are synovial and are called the **carpometacarpal joints**.

The thumb metacarpal articulates with the trapezium and forms a synovial joint which has its own capsule and synovial membrane. This is necessary since the thumb is so mobile. When the hand in the anatomical position, the palmar surface of the thumb does not face directly forwards like the fingers. This is because the thumb metacarpal sits on the trapezium in a different orientation. Because of this difference in orientation the movements of the thumb also take place in different planes to those of the fingers. Thus to *flex* the thumb it must be moved medially and for *extension* it should move laterally (Fig. 3.15). Adduction is a movement towards the palm and abduction a movement away from it (Fig. 3.16). A combination of these four movements is circumduction of the thumb. Perhaps the most important movement at the thumb carpometacarpal joint is a rotation that brings the thumb around into a position where the tip of the thumb can be placed against the tip of a finger (Fig. 3.17). This movement is called **opposition**.

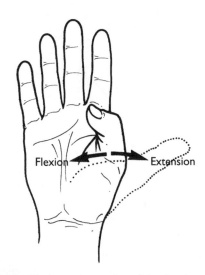

Figure 3.15 Flexion and extension of the thumb at the carpometacarpal joint.

This precision type of movement is used to hold and manipulate things and in picking up small objects.

The other carpometacarpal joints are not as mobile as the thumb. In fact the joints between the finger metacarpals and the carpal bones share the same synovial cavity with the midcarpal joints. The index metacarpal articulates mainly with the trapezoid, the middle metacarpal with the capitate, and the ring and little finger metacarpals with the hamate (Fig. 3.9). There is very little movement at these joints but the

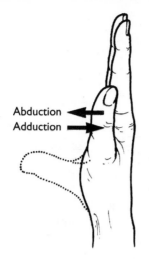

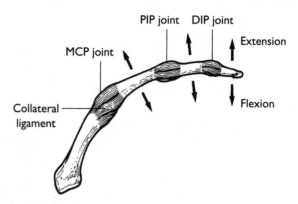

Figure 3.18 The MCP, PIP and DIP joints of the finger. The arrows indicate that flexion and extension can occur at each of these joints.

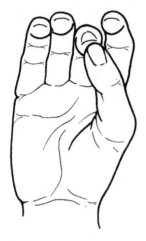

Figure 3.16 Abduction and adduction of the thumb.

Figure 3.17 Opposition of the thumb, in this case with the tip of the middle finger.

interphalangeal joints and those between the middle and distal phalanges are the **distal interphalangeal joints.** These names are rather long to pronounce and much longer to write down! It is much easier to abbreviate them as MCP, PIP and DIP joints (Fig. 3.18). This is a useful shorthand when recording findings of, for example, a clinical examination of the fingers. The movements of the thumb and fingers are extremely important in everyday life. Many activities that are taken for granted cannot be performed if the thumb or fingers become immobile. The movements at the MCP joints are different from those at the IP joints.

The MCP joints are condyloid and therefore allow **flexion, extension, abduction** and **adduction,** and the little finger metacarpal can be flexed and rotated (opposed) to increase the cupping of the palm of the hand. The bases of the finger metacarpals are united by strong ligaments.

The bony framework of the fingers and thumb is made up of small cylindrical bones called **phalanges** (Fig. 3.9). Each finger has three phalanges, a **proximal,** a **middle** and a **distal phalanx,** whilst the thumb has only a **proximal** and a **distal phalanx.** The phalanges are united by synovial joints to the heads of the metacarpals and to each other. The articulations with the metacarpal heads are called **metacarpophalangeal joints** and those between phalanges are **interphalangeal joints.** The interphalangeal joints between the proximal and middle phalanges are the **proximal**

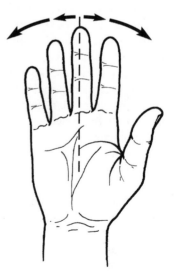

Figure 3.19 Deviation away from the midline of the hand during abduction of the fingers.

combination movement of **circumduction** (but not rotation in the long axis of the bone). A word of explanation is needed about the terms adduction and abduction when applied to the MCP joints. When describing the MCP joints of the **fingers**, abduction means deviation away from the midline of the hand and adduction towards that line (Fig. 3.19). This is a rather unsatisfactory nomenclature when applied clinically (see p. 53). Abduction and adduction of the **thumb** follows the pattern shown in Figure 3.16, abduction being a movement away from the palm and adduction towards the palm.

The IP joints are hinge joints and therefore allow only **flexion** and **extension** (Figs 3.15 and 3.18). Try now to go through the movements of each MCP and IP joint on your own hand. Learn carefully the capabilities and limitations of each of these joints.

The capsules of all the MCP and IP joints are strengthened by collateral ligaments on either side. Their palmar surfaces are also strengthened by so-called palmar ligaments. Sometimes small **sesamoid bones** are developed in these palmar ligaments, especially in the palmar ligament of the MCP joint of the thumb.

chapter
4

The Front of the Forearm and Palm of the Hand

General arrangement of the muscles of the forearm and hand

Broadly speaking, the muscles of the forearm and hand can be conveniently divided into two groups. The muscles and tendons of the **front of the forearm** run into the **palmar surface of the wrist** and the **palm of the hand**. The muscles of the **back of the forearm** run to the **back of the wrist** and the **dorsum of the hand**. The functions of these muscles are also grouped together so that the muscles on the **front** of the forearm are the **pronators** of the forearm and the **flexors** of the wrist and digits. The muscles on the **back** of the forearm, however, are the **supinators** of the forearm and the **extensors** of the wrist and digits. This basic concept is a very helpful thing to remember. There is, in fact, only one exception to this pattern. One extensor muscle has retained its 'extensor' nerve supply but has come to function as a flexor.

Both flexor and extensor compartments are arranged in **superficial** and **deep** layers. Each superficial stratum arises from an **epicondyle of the humerus** and each deep stratum from the **forearm bones and interosseous membrane**. Thus on the front of the forearm the **superficial** muscles arise from the **medial epicondyle** and the **deep** muscles from the forearm bones and interosseous membrane, whilst on the back the **superficial** muscles arise from the **lateral epicondyle** and the **deep** muscles from the back of the forearm bones and interosseous membrane.

Note in passing that the pronators and supinators always **arise** from a 'stable' bone, i.e. the ulna or humerus, and never from the radius. With these general thoughts in mind the remainder of this chapter and Chapter 5 divide our study of the forearm and hand into two parts. First, we will study the front of the forearm and palm of the hand and then in Chapter 5 we will study the back of the forearm and of the hand. We can then consider how all of these structures fulfil their primary goal of bringing about movements of the fingers and thumb.

The front of the forearm and the palm of the hand

The muscles on the front of the forearm are arranged in **superficial** and **deep** layers. There are five muscles in the superficial stratum and they arise in part or wholly from a common origin on the **medial epicondyle** of the humerus (Fig. 4.1). Functionally, they are the **pronators** of the forearm and the **flexors** of the wrist, fingers and thumb. One extra muscle is seen on the radial side of the front of the forearm. It originally belonged to the extensor muscle mass of the forearm and indeed is supplied by the extensor nerve (radial). However, it has migrated around the front to take up a function of a flexor of the **elbow**. (It does not extend into the wrist.) This muscle is called the **brachioradialis** and is the 'exception' we referred to above.

Consider first the four muscles that are concerned with pronation of the forearm and flexion of the wrist. Do not be disturbed by the names – the Latin nomenclature simply describes the function of the

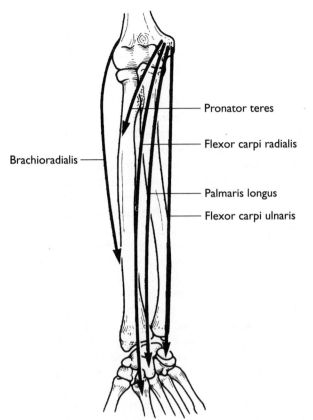

Figure 4.1 The five superficial muscles on the front of the forearm.

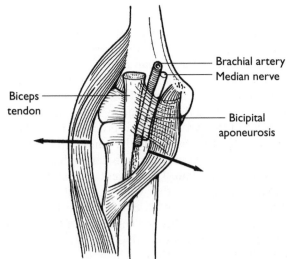

Figure 4.2 The structures of the cubital fossa.

muscles. They are called the **pronator teres** (round-bodied muscle for pronating the forearm) and the **flexor carpi radialis** (the flexor of the radial side of the wrist). It might help you to repeat these names several times until you become familiar with them: anatomy is after all only like learning another 'language'!

Notice in Figure 4.1 that the pronator teres and brachioradialis converge towards one another in the forearm. The intermuscular space between them, which lies in front of the elbow, is called the **cubital fossa**. It is said to be a 'triangular' intermuscular interval bounded by these two muscles and an imaginary line drawn between the two epicondyles of the humerus (Fig. 4.2).

Almost all of the **pronator teres** arises from the common origin on the medial epicondyle of the humerus. In fact a small slip of muscle arises from the coronoid process of the ulna but this is of little importance. The muscle forms the medial border of the **cubital fossa** as it passes to its insertion on the lateral side of the radius (Fig. 4.3). Its action is to

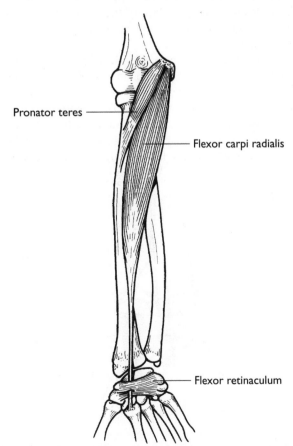

Figure 4.3 Pronator teres and flexor carpi radialis.

pronate the forearm. Since, however, it arises from the humerus and is inserted into the forearm, it can also act as a weak flexor of the elbow joint. The muscle is supplied by the **median nerve**.

The **flexor carpi radialis** also arises from the common flexor origin. In the distal part of the forearm the muscle belly gives rise to a tendon which passes over the front of the wrist joint and proceeds to its destination into the base of the index metacarpal (Fig. 4.3). It is held in place by a fibrous band called the **flexor retinaculum**. This prevents the tendon from springing away from the wrist during flexion. The retinaculum is attached on either side to the carpal bones and thus converts the concavity of the carpus into an **osseofascial tunnel** (Fig. 4.4). The retinaculum helps to maintain the concavity of the carpus as well as holding down the tendons. In fact, the function of holding down tendons has probably been over-emphasized in the past. The flexor carpi radialis passes through the tunnel in a groove on the trapezium to its destination into the base of the index metacarpal. Fibres from the deep surface of the retinaculum convert this groove into a kind of 'private' tunnel for the tendon.

Another important principle must be learned now. When tendons pass through an osseofascial tunnel they need to be surrounded by a lubricating sheath to reduce friction to a minimum. The sheath is formed from two tubes of synovial membrane, (exactly the same as that found in synovial joints). The inner tube is closely applied to the tendon and the outer tube to the tunnel wall. The two tubes are continuous with each other proximally and distally so that between them is a closed potential space containing only a film of lubricating synovial fluid (Fig. 4.5).

The flexor carpi radialis can bring about **flexion** and **abduction** at the wrist joint. It is supplied by the **median nerve**. The **palmaris longus** is an inconsistent, delicate muscle which arises from the common flexor origin and is inserted into the dense fascia of the palm of the hand. It does not pass through the osseofascial tunnel, but rather travels over the surface of the flexor retinaculum. It therefore has no need of a synovial sheath. It is supplied by the **median nerve** and is a weak **flexor** of the wrist (Fig. 4.6).

The **flexor carpi ulnaris** arises from the common origin on the medial epicondyle and from the olecranon and posterior border of the ulna. The detail of its origin is best seen from the posterior aspect of the elbow (Fig. 4.7). The muscle passes down the forearm and becomes tendinous (Fig. 4.6). In the region of the triquetrum the tendon contains a sesamoid bone called the **pisiform**. This is united to the surface of the triquetrum by a synovial joint. The tendon finally inserts into the hook of the hamate and the fifth metacarpal by means of the pisohamate and pisometacarpal ligaments. The detail of the insertion of the flexor carpi ulnaris is shown in Figure 4.8.

The tendon of the flexor carpi ulnaris does not therefore pass through the osseofascial tunnel at the wrist and so has no need of a synovial sheath. It can **flex** and **adduct** the wrist joint. Since it passes between the humerus and the wrist it also spans the elbow joint and is therefore a weak flexor of this joint. The pisiform bone is often described as being one of the carpal bones; it is more logical, however, to think of it as a sesamoid in the tendon of the flexor carpi ulnaris. It can be enucleated without altering the

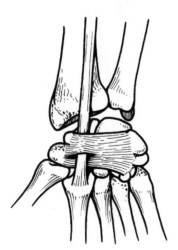

Figure 4.4   The flexor retinaculum and the tendon of flexor carpi radialis.

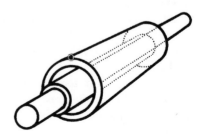

Figure 4.5   Two continuous layers of a synovial sheath surround each tendon and enclose a potential space filled only with a film of synovial fluid.

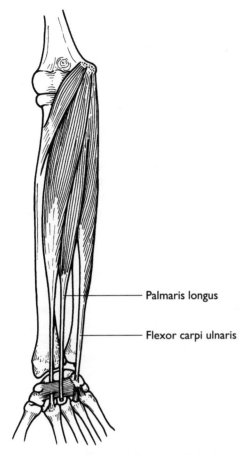

Figure 4.6 Palmaris longus and flexor carpi ulnaris.

Palmaris longus

Flexor carpi ulnaris

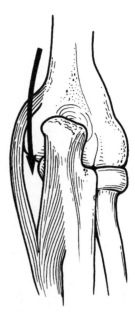

Figure 4.7 The two origins of flexor carpi ulnaris seen from the posterior aspect of the elbow. The arrow indicates the path of the ulnar nerve as it negotiates the elbow region.

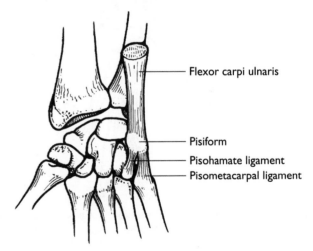

Flexor carpi ulnaris

Pisiform

Pisohamate ligament

Pisometacarpal ligament

Figure 4.8 Details of the insertion of flexor carpi ulnaris into the pisiform and hamate and base of the 5th metacarpal.

function of the ulnaris tendon. The nerve supply to the muscle is the **ulnar nerve**.

Look now at Figure 4.6. The four muscles described form a sort of 'roof' over the deeper structures. To see the **fifth** member of the superficial group the muscles of the 'roof' have to be removed (Fig. 4.9). The fifth member of the superficial group therefore lies a little deeper than the other members. It is concerned with producing **flexion of the four fingers** and is therefore called the **flexor digitorum superficialis**.

This muscle is large and arises from the **humerus**, the **ulna** and the **radius**. Learn this muscle carefully and learn to find it in dissected specimens for it is the 'key' to the neurovascular relations in the forearm. The humeroulnar head arises from the common origin of the humerus and from the coronoid process of the ulna (Fig. 4.9). The radial head arises from the anterior border of the radius. Between these origins is a fibrous arch. The large muscle belly gives rise to

four tendons in the lower reaches of the forearm. These tendons pass to the four fingers.

As the tendons pass over the wrist they pass through the osseofascial tunnel and so need to be surrounded by a synovial sheath. They are grouped in pairs in this region, the tendons to the ring and middle fingers being superficial to those of the index and little fingers. On passing into the palm of the hand they flatten out into a single row. The synovial sheath

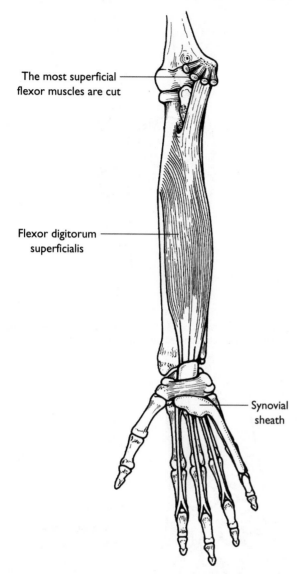

Figure 4.9   The fifth member of the superficial group of flexor muscles lies beneath the other four and is the flexor digitorum superficialis.

The most superficial flexor muscles are cut

Flexor digitorum superficialis

Synovial sheath

flexor sheaths (Fig. 4.10). Thus they pass through an osseofascial tunnel along the digits. The fibrous sheaths are attached to the margins of the phalanges and their distal ends fuse with the terminal phalanx. As the tendons pass in this way they once again become surrounded by lubricating synovial sheaths. Penetrating injuries, therefore, of the palmar aspects of the fingers can introduce infection into the synovial sheaths in the osseofascial tunnels of the finger. In the case of the little finger this sheath is continuous with the common sheath that surrounds the tendons as they pass through the osseofascial tunnel of the wrist and a more widespread synovial sheath infection may be anticipated.

The blood supply to the tendons is also important since, if it is cut off during severe infection of the hand or fingers, the tendons will slough and rupture. In the osseofascial tunnel of the wrist the blood vessels are able to enter quite simply since the tendons invaginate the synovial sheath (Fig. 4.11). In the osseofascial tunnels of the fingers, local vessels need to pierce the synovial sheaths because here the sheaths completely surround the tendons. As the blood vessels pass to the tendons they are surrounded by a little fibrous tissue. The blood vessels and their surrounding fibrous tissue are called **vincula** (Fig. 4.12). Those that supply the tendon near its insertion are obviously short and, therefore, called vincula brevia; others that are longer are called vincula longa.

The nerve supply to the flexor digitorum superficialis muscle is the **median nerve**. The muscle, clearly, is a flexor of the metacarpophalangeal and proximal interphalangeal joints of the fingers. Now, with

of the little finger tendon continues into the little finger but the common sheath surrounding the other three ends just distal to the osseofascial tunnel in the palm. The pattern of synovial sheaths, however, is always variable. The sheaths are important clinically if penetrating wounds of the hand allow infection to enter the sheaths.

The tendons of the superficialis split near their terminations and insert into the middle phalanges of the fingers (Fig. 4.9). As they pass along the palmar surfaces of the fingers, they are held in place by **fibrous**

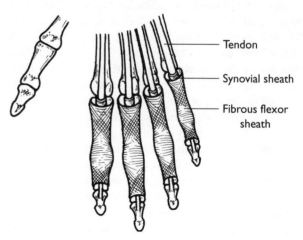

Tendon

Synovial sheath

Fibrous flexor sheath

Figure 4.10   Fibrous flexor sheaths hold the flexor tendons of the fingers in place.

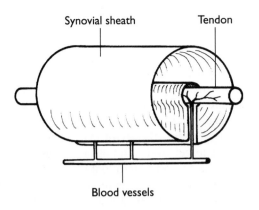

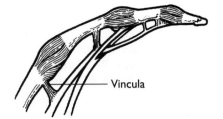

Figure 4.12 In the osseofascial tunnels surrounding the fingers, blood vessels need to pierce the synovial sheaths to gain access to the tendons.

Figure 4.11 In the wrist, blood vessels enter tendons along the path of invagination of the tendons into the synovial sheath.

the aid of Figure 4.13, review the insertions of the muscles of the superficial stratum which insert into the wrist and fingers.

Attention may now be turned to the **deep** layer of muscles on the front of the forearm. These three

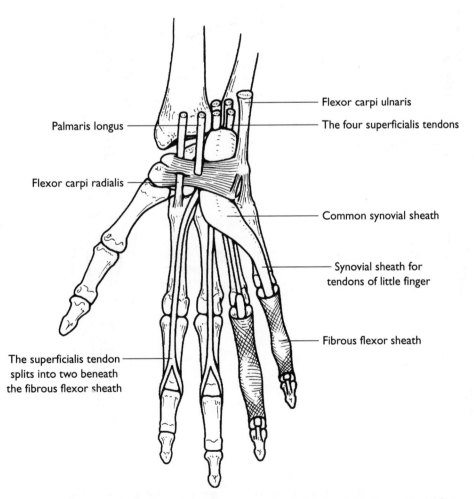

Figure 4.13 The muscles of the superficial group of the flexor compartment that insert into the wrist and fingers.

muscles arise from and are in contact with the forearm bones and interosseous membrane. They are the **pronator quadratus** (quadrilaterally shaped pronator of the forearm), the **flexor pollicis longus** (a long flexor for the thumb) and the **flexor digitorum profundus** (a deeply placed flexor for the four fingers). Their outlines are represented by Figure 4.14.

The muscles of the superficial stratum, with the exception of the flexor carpi ulnaris, were supplied by the median nerve. Similarly, the three muscles of the deep stratum are supplied by a branch of the **median nerve** called the **anterior interosseous nerve**. The ulnar side of the flexor digitorum profundus, however, also receives supply from the **ulnar** nerve.

The **pronator quadratus** arises from the lower quarter of the ulna and passes obliquely across to the radius. As its name implies it is a pronator of the forearm and is supplied by the anterior interosseous nerve (Fig. 4.15).

The **flexor pollicis longus** arises from the radial side of the forearm, that is from the front of the radius and adjacent interosseous membrane. Above the wrist its muscular belly gives rise to a tendon which, like those of the fingers, passes through the osseofascial tunnel at the wrist to get to the thumb. It passes along the thumb to insert into the terminal phalanx. Its action is therefore to flex all the joints of the thumb. It is held against the thumb by a fibrous flexor sheath. As the tendon passes through the osseofascial tunnel of the wrist and the fibrous sheath it is surrounded by a synovial sheath (Fig. 4.15). The muscle is supplied by the **anterior interosseous nerve**.

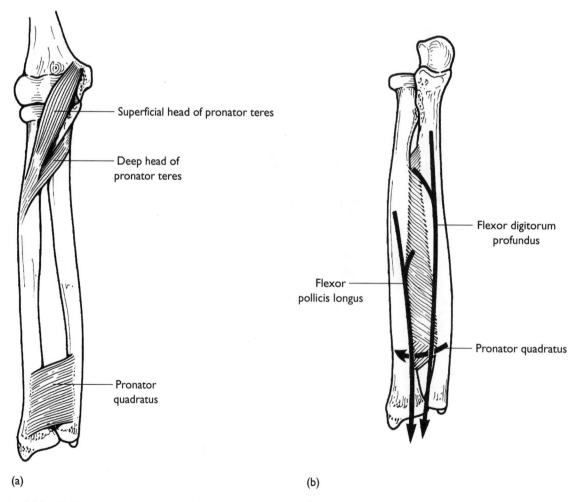

(a)   (b)

Figure 4.14   (a) The two pronator muscles of the forearm shown together. (b) The three muscles in the deep layer on the front of the forearm.

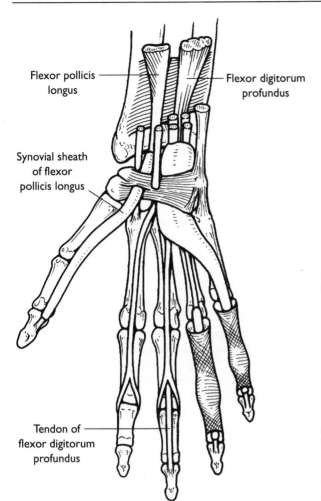

Figure 4.15 The relationship of flexor pollicis longus and flexor digitorum profundus to the superficial tendons and muscles in the wrist and hand.

The **flexor digitorum profundus** forms a large fleshy mass which arises from the anterior and medial surfaces of the ulna and adjacent interosseous membrane (Fig. 4.14). Four tendons arise from the fleshy belly and pass through the osseofascial tunnel at the wrist. Note that here they share the common synovial sheath with the tendons of flexor digitorum superficialis. The tendons lie deep to those of the superficialis and proceed to the fingers in this manner. They enter the fibrous flexor sheaths of the fingers deep to the superficialis tendons. They are destined to be inserted into the **terminal phalanges**, and to get there they slip through the split superficialis tendon (Figs 4.16 & 4.17). The muscle therefore produces flexion of both interphalangeal joints and of the metacarpophalangeal joints of the fingers.

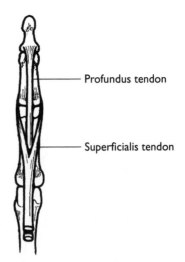

Figure 4.16 The profundus tendon pierces the superficialis tendon.

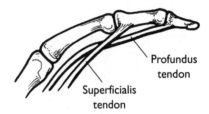

Figure 4.17 The profundus tendon continues on, to insert into the terminal phalanx.

While in the fibrous flexor tunnels of the fingers the tendons are surrounded by synovial sheath. The muscle is supplied by the **anterior interosseous nerve** but some of the more medial fibres receive a supply from the **ulnar nerve**. Review, with the help of Figure 4.18, the positions of synovial sheaths in the fingers and wrist. They occur wherever tendons pass through osseofascial tunnels. Penetrating wounds in these areas are potentially dangerous since they may introduce infection which can spread rapidly along the sheaths. Accumulation of pus in the sheaths will increase the pressure and the swelling may affect the blood supply of the tendons, which may slough and rupture. Inflammation of synovial sheaths around tendons is called **tenosynovitis**.

The short muscles acting on the fingers and thumb

The time has now come to look in detail at the movements which occur in the thumb and fingers. It takes

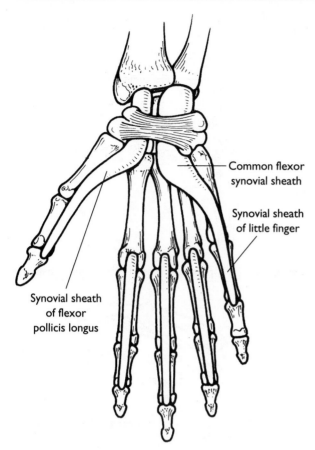

Figure 4.18 The position and arrangement of the synovial sheaths of the flexor tendons in the wrist and fingers.

only a few moments of thought to realize how important these movements are. They are vital to almost all daily activities. Loss of function in the fingers or thumb is therefore disabling. The muscles acting on the fingers and thumb arise in the forearm and in the hand itself. Some of them are therefore **long** and some are **short** muscles. The long muscles have already been studied. They are the **flexor digitorum superficialis** and **profundus** and the **flexor pollicis longus**. Review these muscles once again. They are responsible for flexion of the fingers and thumb.

Turn your attention to the *short* muscles that act on the fingers and thumb. They arise in the palm of the hand. With a complete knowledge of these long and short muscles you will be in a position to understand the functional anatomy of the fingers and thumb. The **interosseous muscles** are deeply placed between the metacarpal bones. The **thenar muscles** form the fleshy mass on the palmar surface of the thumb metacarpal, and the **hypothenar muscles** the

mass on the palmar surface of the little finger metacarpal. Four other short muscles that are associated with the profundus tendons in the palm also need to be studied. Before proceeding to study these **short muscles** be sure that you understand the movements that can occur in the **metacarpophalangeal joints** and in the **interphalangeal joints**. The latter present no problem since the only movements are **flexion** and **extension**. However, the movements of the metacarpophalangeal joints do present certain difficulties of a nomenclatural nature.

Classically the MCP joints are said to be capable of **flexion, extension, abduction** and **adduction**. Flexion and extension are clear, but do not forget that the thumb flexes and extends in a plane at right angles to the other fingers (see p. 39). The main stumbling block to understanding the function of the digits is the definitions of **abduction** and **adduction**. Abduction and adduction are described as movements away from and towards the **midline of the hand**. The midline is defined as a line that passes through the middle finger (Fig. 4.19). Learn the muscles and their actions according to this classical description first, but then go one step further in your study. Recognize that the functional division of the hand in a power grip is between the thumb and thenar eminence on the one

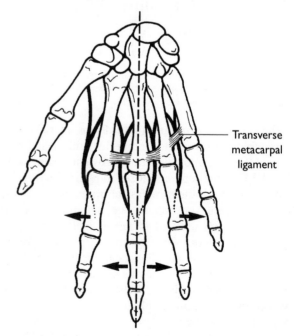

Figure 4.19 A line through the middle finger defines the midline of the hand. Abduction (arrows) and adduction are movements away from and towards the midline respectively.

side and the fingers and palm on the other. You have only to grasp any object to verify this.

The **interosseous muscles** arise from the metacarpal bones. They are, quite naturally, divided into two sets, four **dorsal** muscles and four **palmar** muscles. The four dorsal interosseous muscles arise from adjacent sides of the metacarpals (Fig. 4.19). The muscles give way to tendons which pass deep to the ligaments uniting the metacarpal heads of the index, middle and ring fingers and pass on to the **dorsum** of the fingers. Here on the dorsum they are inserted into the extensor **tendon** of that finger.

According to the classical definition, therefore, their action is to **abduct** the **middle three digits** (index, middle and ring fingers). An easy way to remember this is to use the formula DAB₃ (dorsal abduct middle three digits). The dorsal interossei have an additional function. Looked at from the side, as in Figure 4.20, it can be imagined that they might be able to flex the metacarpophalangeal joint. Since they insert into the extensor tendon, they would also extend the interphalangeal joints. Put more simply, *they are able to flex a straight finger.* In summary, the dorsal interossei act on the middle three digits they can abduct these digits at the MCP joints and they can also flex these joints and straighten the IP joints.

The four palmar interosseous muscles arise from the palmar aspects of the metacarpals. The middle metacarpal has no need for an adductor since either of its abductors can perform this function anyway. Each palmar interosseous gives rise to a tendon that passes deep to the metacarpal ligaments to reach the dorsum of the corresponding digit (Fig. 4.21). Their insertion is into the extensor tendon as in the case of the dorsal muscles. They **adduct** or close the thumb, index, ring and little fingers to the midline of the palm. This action is not needed for the middle finger

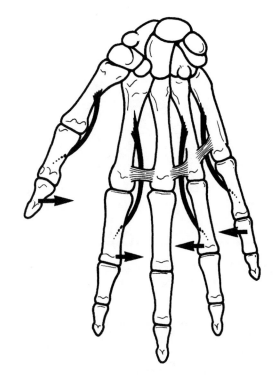

Figure 4.21 Each palmar interosseous muscle gives rise to a tendon which passes deep to the metacarpal ligament to reach the back of the corresponding digit.

since it can be taken to the midline by its dorsal muscles. The 'formula' to aid the memory for these muscles and their action is PAD (palmar adduct). Once again notice that these muscles can also flex the straight digit. The first palmar interosseous is a very small slip of muscle; it is given a different name in some textbooks, but it is easier to remember that there are four dorsal and four palmar interossei.

All MCP joints are capable of **abduction** and **adduction** but it can be seen that the interossei do not completely fulfil these functions. Certain other muscles are needed for movement of the thumb and little finger. The first palmar interosseous is slender and cannot adduct the thumb strongly enough. Situated deep in the palm, therefore, we find a special adductor for the thumb called the **adductor pollicis** (Fig. 4.22) which can almost be thought of as a very large palmar interosseous muscle. The **adductor pollicis** arises in the form of two heads from the palmar surfaces of the second and third metacarpals. The two heads unite and insert into the medial side of the base of the proximal phalanx of the thumb. The muscle is on a more superficial plane to the first dorsal interosseous and

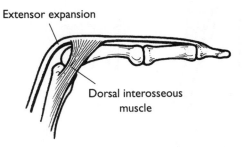

Figure 4.20 The dorsal interossei are able to extend the interphalangeal joints and flex the metacarpophalangeal joint; put more simply, they can flex a straight finger.

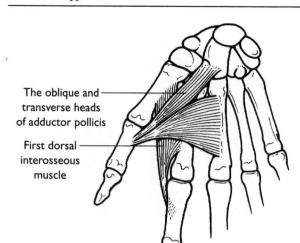

The oblique and transverse heads of adductor pollicis

First dorsal interosseous muscle

Figure 4.22 The two heads of adductor pollicis with the first dorsal interosseous muscle posterior to it.

first palmar interosseous muscles. The muscle is a powerful **adductor** of the thumb at the MCP joint. All the interosseous muscles and the adductor pollicis are supplied by the **ulnar nerve**.

In addition to the adductor pollicis, the thumb has several other small muscles. These are grouped on the palmar surface of the first metacarpal where they are seen as a fleshy mass. This mass is known as the the-

nar eminence and the muscles are called the **thenar muscles**. The group includes three muscles: the **abductor pollicis brevis**, the **flexor pollicis brevis** and the **opponens pollicis**. All three muscles arise from the lateral aspect of the flexor retinaculum and the scaphoid and trapezium where their origins blend (Fig. 4.23).

The flexor and abductor are inserted into the lateral side of the base of the proximal phalanx of the thumb. As their names suggest they flex and abduct the thumb at its MCP joint. The opponens, however, lies on a deeper plane and is inserted into the shaft of the thumb metacarpal. It can rotate the shaft of the thumb metacarpal so that the palmar surface of the thumb faces the palmar surface of the fingers. This movement is called opposition. The three short muscles of the thumb are supplied by the **median nerve**.

Three similar muscles are found on the palmar surface of the little finger metacarpal. They are the **abductor digiti minimi**, the **flexor digiti minimi** and, on a deeper plane, the **opponens digiti minimi** (Fig. 4.23). All three muscles arise from the pisiform and hook of the hamate where their origin blends with the medial end of the flexor retinaculum. The flexor and abductor are inserted into the base of the proximal phalanx of the little finger and their actions

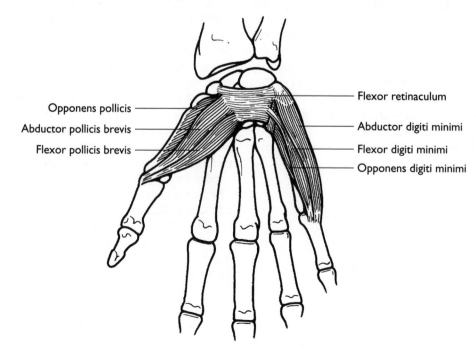

Opponens pollicis

Abductor pollicis brevis

Flexor pollicis brevis

Flexor retinaculum

Abductor digiti minimi

Flexor digiti minimi

Opponens digiti minimi

Figure 4.23 The muscles of the thenar and hypothenar eminence.

are flexion and abduction of the little finger at the MCP joint. The opponens, like that of the thumb, inserts into the outer aspect of the shaft of the fifth metacarpal and is able to rotate the shaft of that bone, so deepening the cup of the palm. All three muscles are supplied by the **ulnar nerve.**

A small subcutaneous muscle is found overlying the hypothenar muscles. It arises from the flexor retinaculum and is inserted into the skin on the ulnar border of the palm. It is called the **palmaris brevis** and puckers the skin in this region, so deepening slightly the cup of the palm. It is also supplied by the **ulnar nerve.**

Now go through what you have already learned about the muscles that act on the thumb and fingers. The long tendons that flex the fingers are those of the flexor digitorum superficialis and profundus. Superficialis flexes the PIP and MCP joints but the profundus also flexes the DIP joints. The flexor pollicis longus flexes the IP and MCP joints of the thumb. Flexion of the thumb and little finger at the MCP joints is aided by the small flexor pollicis brevis and flexor digiti minimi muscles respectively. The interosseus muscles can flex the MCP joints while keeping the IP joints extended.   Now examine the movements of abduction and adduction and of opposition. A look at Figure 4.24 will show you that all digits are capable of abduction away from and adduction towards the midline. This movement takes place at the **MCP joints.** Much of it is performed by the **interosseous muscles,**

but the thumb and little finger have additional specialized muscles. In the case of the thumb the weak adductor, first palmar interosseous, is strengthened by the **adductor pollicis** and abduction is performed by the **abductor pollicis brevis.** In the little finger abduction is performed by the **abductor digiti minimi.**

Look at Figure 4.25. It is a drawing of a hand about to grip a cylindrical object. Notice that the position of the fingers during function, i.e. when anything is held in the hand or between the fingers and thumb, is not arranged around the middle finger. The functional division of the hand is between thumb and thenar eminence on one side, and the fingers, palm and hypothenar eminence on the other. The terms adduction and abduction now become difficult to apply to these simple functional movements. In this situation it makes much more sense to replace these terms with others that describe these movements more meaningfully.

Movements of the MCP joints are therefore better described as flexion, extension, **radial deviation** and **ulnar deviation.** Look once again at Figure 4.25. The fingers are all swung together towards the ulnar side of the limb. This deviation occurs at the MCP joints and is produced by certain interossei and the abductor digiti minimi. The thumb deviates towards the radial side and this is produced by the abductor pollicis

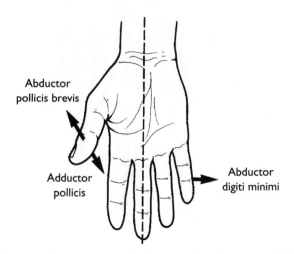

Figure 4.24 Abduction and adduction take place at the MCP joints. The interossei manage most of this but the thumb and little finger have additional muscles (shown in the figure) acting on them.

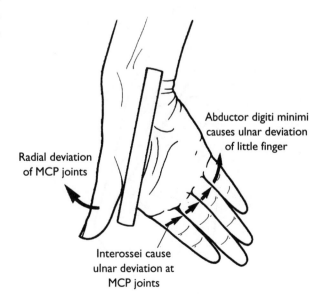

Figure 4.25 In this situation, where the hand is about to grip a cylindrical object, functional division of the hand is between the thumb and thenar eminence on the one side and the fingers, palm and hypothenar eminence on the other side.

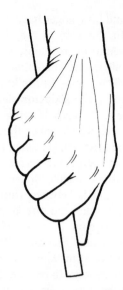

Figure 4.26 Notice the ulnar deviation at the finger MCP joints and radial deviation at the thumb MCP joint.

brevis. With the MCP joints in this position of function, the opponens pollicis and opponens digiti minimi rotate the first and fifth metacarpals so that the palmar surface of the thumb faces the palmar surfaces of the fingers and the palm is cupped. The long flexors may now curl the thumb and fingers around the object and grip it firmly in a 'power grip'.

Hold a cylindrical object such as the handle of a hammer in the hand. Look at the position of the MCP

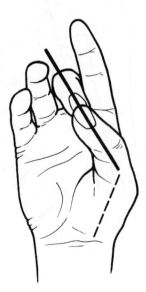

Figure 4.27 In opposition, the thumb MCP joint is radially deviated and the finger MCP joint is ulnar deviated.

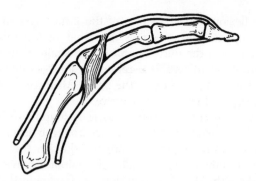

Figure 4.28 Four lumbrical muscles arise from the radial side of the profundus tendons in the palm and insert with the interossei into the corresponding extensor tendon.

joints of the fingers and thumb. The finger joints are ulnar deviated and the thumb radially deviated (Fig. 4.26). The same pattern of deviation may be seen if you oppose the thumb pad to the little finger pad in a 'precision grip' (Fig. 4.27). Notice again the deviation at the two MCP joints. Thus, during function, the MCP joints are never used as though there were a midline: fingers act together and the thumb acts by itself.

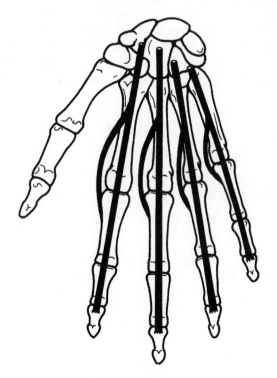

Figure 4.29 The four lumbrical muscles each arise from tendons and insert into tendons on the radial side of the fingers.

Four delicate muscles now need to be mentioned. They are called the **lumbrical muscles**. They arise from the radial side of the profundus tendons in the palm, pass to the dorsum of the corresponding finger and insert with the interossei into the extensor tendon. They thus **arise from tendons** and are inserted into **tendons** (Figs 4.28 & 4.29). The lumbricals, like the interossei, can flex the straight finger. However, unlike the interossei, they cannot abduct or adduct the fingers. By passing from flexor to extensor tendons they integrate the actions of these by altering tension in the tendons and so allowing a delicate and fine coordination in the movements of the fingers. The lateral two lumbricals are supplied by the **median nerve** and the medial two by the **ulnar nerve**. Figure 4.30 shows a finger with each of its associated tendons and muscles.

The fascia investing the muscles in the palm is fairly strong. On either side, fascia invests the **thenar** and **hypothenar** muscle masses (Fig. 4.31). Between these two raised eminences, in the palm of the hand beneath the skin, is a very strong fascial sheet. This is called the **palmar aponeurosis**. It is more or less triangular in shape, the apex being fused with the fibres of the flexor retinaculum. At this point the tendon of the palmaris longus gains insertion into it. The base of the aponeurosis divides into four fascial processes at the roots of the fingers. Here they fuse with the fibrous sheaths for the flexor tendons. If the palmar aponeurosis is removed, as in Figure 4.32, an **intermediate compartment** of the palm can be seen. This contains the tendons of the superficialis and profundus, blood vessels and some nerves. In the depths the adductor pollicis muscle can be seen covered with fascia.

Thus there are then four 'fascial compartments' in the palm: lateral and medial compartments containing the thenar and hypothenar muscles, an intermediate compartment roofed by the palmar aponeurosis and containing important tendons and nerves, and a deeper compartment containing the adductor pollicis muscle. Fascial coverings are important only if they limit the spread of infection or malignant disease. In the case of the fascial compartments of the palm, they are useful to know since infections in the palm may be limited to one or other of these potential spaces.

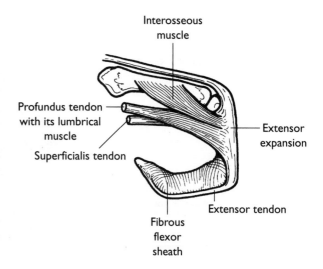

Figure 4.30 The tendons, interossei and associated lumbrical muscle of a finger.

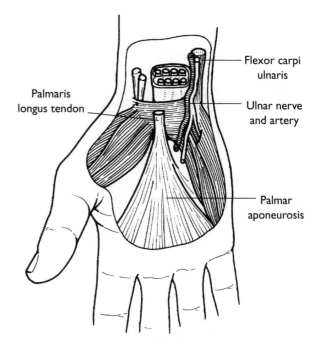

Figure 4.31 The palmar aponeurosis and the thenar and hypothenar eminences.

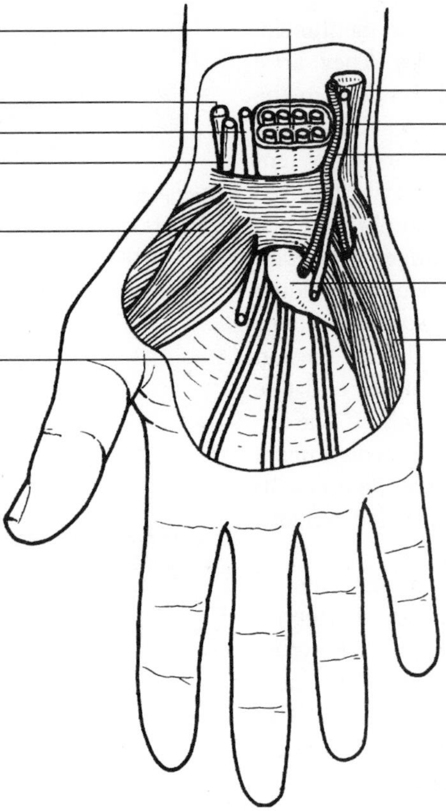

Superficialis and profundus tendons

Flexor pollicis longus

Median nerve

Flexor carpi radialis

Thenar eminence

Lateral fascial septum covering adductor pollicis

Flexor carpi ulnaris

Ulnar nerve

Ulnar artery

Common synovial sheath

Hypothenar eminence

Figure 4.32   The intermediate compartment of the palm beneath the palmar aponeurosis contains the superficialis and profundus tendons as well as blood vessels and nerves.

The Back of the Forearm and Back of the Hand

We will now study the muscles on the back of the forearm and back of the hand. They are all 'long' muscles that arise from the arm and pass down into the back of the wrist and back of the hand. There are no 'short' muscles arising from the back of the hand itself, as was the case in the palm.

Like the flexor muscles on the front of the forearm, the extensor muscles on the back may also be conveniently divided into **superficial** and **deep groups**. The superficial group arises from the **lateral epicondyle** of the humerus and the **deep group** from the **forearm bones** and **interosseous membrane**. (Compare this with the flexor arrangement in Figures 4.1 and 4.14.) Whereas the muscles of the front of the forearm were pronators or flexors, those of the back are functionally **supinators** or **extensors**. Although there are more muscles on the dorsum, their pattern is very simple. Figure 5.1 shows the pattern of the superficial group of muscles.

The first muscle to note once again is the **anconeus**. This small triangular sheet passes from the lateral epicondyle to the olecranon. It can pull on the upper end of the ulna and cause some movement of this bone while pronation and supination are underway. It is supplied by a branch from the radial nerve. More important are the **two radial extensors of the wrist** and the **ulnar extensor of the wrist**. These are named the **extensor carpi radialis longus** and **brevis** and the **extensor carpi ulnaris**.

As the long tendons pass into the wrist and hand they are held against the distal forearm by a thickening in the deep fascia called the **extensor retinaculum**. This bridge of fascia passes between the styloid region of the ulna and triquetrum to the lower end of the

radius. Unlike the flexor osseofascial tunnel, that beneath the extensor retinaculum is divided up by five septa that pass on to the radius and ulna, so making six small osseofascial compartments. The tendons on

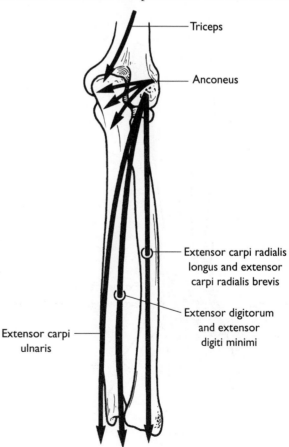

Figure 5.1 The superficial group of muscles on the back of the forearm and hand.

the back of the wrist pass through these tunnels as a single row of tendons. Naturally, as they pass through their respective osseofascial tunnel they are surrounded by a synovial sheath. There is no virtue in remembering the numbers of these tunnels.

The **extensor carpi radialis longus** and **brevis** both arise from the region of the lateral epicondyle and pass down through a tunnel underneath the extensor retinaculum (Fig. 5.2). The longus gains insertion into the base of the second metacarpal (like the flexor carpi radialis). The brevis is inserted into the base of the third metacarpal. The longus is supplied by the radial nerve itself and the brevis by its deep branch. They both **extend** the wrist and since they act on the radial side can also **abduct** it.

The **extensor carpi ulnaris** arises from the lateral epicondyle. Its tendon passes distally over the lower end of the ulna, through the most medial compartment of the extensor retinaculum, to reach the base of the fifth metacarpal. The muscle is supplied by the

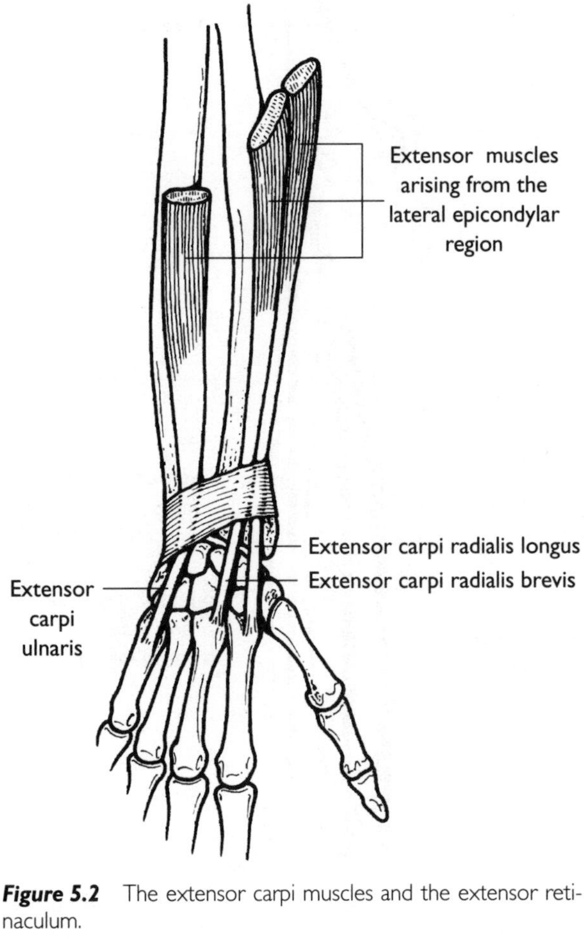

posterior interosseous branch of the radial nerve and it can **extend** and **adduct** the wrist.

Let us pause at this moment to consider the movements of the wrist, since all the muscles acting on this region have now been studied. On the ulnar side of the wrist the flexor muscle is the **flexor carpi ulnaris** and the extensor is the **extensor carpi ulnaris**. Both are inserted into the base of the fifth metacarpal, the flexor by means of the pisometacarpal ligament. Acting together without the radial flexor or extensors they tend to **adduct** the wrist. On the radial side, the flexor is the **flexor carpi radialis** and the extensors are the **extensor carpi radialis longus** and **brevis**. Acting together without the balancing effect of the ulnar muscles they will **abduct** the wrist. Think for a moment of someone using a small hammer in their hand. On the upstroke there is extension of the wrist and also some abduction; during the downstroke there is flexion combined with adduction. Test this integrated type of movement using your own wrist as a model. By acting in sequence these muscles can produce the movement of **circumduction**. Put your wrist through the movements of **flexion, extension, abduction, adduction** and **circumduction**, naming the muscles involved as you do each movement. Extension of the wrist is important not only as a prime movement but also to allow a good flexion grip in the hand. Try to make a tight fist with the wrist fully flexed. There is too much 'slack' in the flexor tendons and the wrist has to be partly extended in order to take up this slack to allow good function of the flexors. Do not forget this when in later years you immobilize an injured forearm in plaster of Paris. The wrist should be fixed in a position of slight extension.

The extensor muscle to the fingers is called the **extensor digitorum**. It arises from the lateral epicondyle and at the wrist passes through an osseofascial compartment beneath the extensor retinaculum (Fig. 5.3). It then divides into four tendons which pass to the four fingers. On the back of the hand these tendons are frequently united by oblique bands which limit to some extent the individual extension of the digits. The little finger and index finger receive an additional small tendon each. The extra tendon to the little finger is called the **extensor digiti minimi**. It arises from the lateral epicondyle and at the wrist it has its own 'private' compartment and synovial sheath. Near the MCP joint it is joined by the extensor digitorum slip to the little finger. The additional tendon to the index finger arises from a muscle called

Figure 5.2 The extensor carpi muscles and the extensor retinaculum.

Labels in figure:
Extensor muscles arising from the lateral epicondylar region
Extensor carpi radialis longus
Extensor carpi radialis brevis
Extensor carpi ulnaris

the **extensor indicis**. This is in fact one of the **deep group** of muscles. It passes through the same osseofascial tunnel as the extensor digitorum at the wrist and joins the tendon of the index finger. The extensor digitorum, extensor indicis and digiti minimi are therefore responsible for extension of the fingers. The section through the extensor retinaculum illustrated in Figure 5.3 shows the details of how the extensor tendons are arranged at the wrist. There is, however, no merit in learning this arrangement by heart. It is sufficient to understand the principle underlying the pattern of these tendons beneath the extensor retinaculum.

As the extensor tendons pass to the fingers they give a small slip to the bases of the proximal phalanges and then flatten out on the surface of the phalanx to form **extensor expansions** (Figs 5.3 and 5.4). Each expansion divides into three slips, the middle being inserted into the base of the middle phalanx and the two collateral slips into the terminal phalanx. It is into these expansions on the surface of the proximal phalanges that the interossei and lumbricals insert. It can be seen from Figure 5.4 that an interosseous tendon inserts as both transverse fibres and as fibres more in line with the extensor tendon. The transverse fibre pull obviously produces the **radial or ulnar devi-**

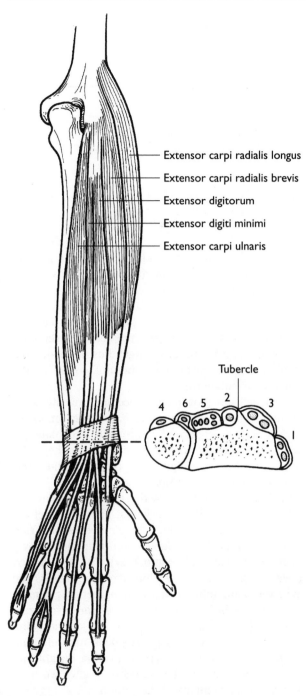

Figure 5.3 In the section through the extensor retinaculum, compartments 1 and 2 contain the extensor and adductors of the thumb, 3 and 4 the wrist extensors, and 5 and 6 the finger extensors. The extensor expansions of extensor digitorum divide into three slips. Two collateral slips pass to the sides of the terminal phalanx and the middle slip runs to the base of the middle phalanx.

Extensor carpi radialis longus
Extensor carpi radialis brevis
Extensor digitorum
Extensor digiti minimi
Extensor carpi ulnaris

Tubercle

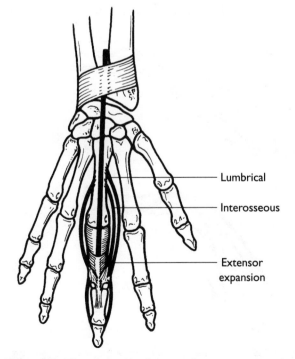

Lumbrical

Interosseous

Extensor expansion

Figure 5.4 The relationships between the extensor expansion and the lumbrical and interossei muscles.

ation (abduction or adduction of classical nomenclature). Pull on the straight fibres will bend the straight finger (flex the MCP and extend the IP joints; Fig. 5.5). The delicate lumbrical tendons on the other hand are inserted mainly in line with the finger and so their main action will be to flex the straight finger.

This is a good time to review the action of muscles on a finger since all the muscles have now been studied. All the extensors are supplied by the posterior interosseous branch of the radial nerve. The movements in the fingers that need to be considered occur in both the MCP and IP joints. There is one other specialized movement associated with the little finger and that is opposition or rotation of the fifth metacarpal. **Flexion** in the MCP joints are produced by the **flexor digitorum superficialis** and **profundus** tendons. **Extension** is produced by the **extensor digitorum** assisted by the **extensor digiti minimi** and **indicis** in the case of the fifth and index fingers. These movements of flexion and extension are gross movements, used, for example, when picking up a case by its handle. The fingers are **extended** by the extensor tendons and then **flexed** as they curl around the handle. There has been pure flexion and extension at the MCP joints. Much more delicate flexion and extension is, however, possible. Take a pencil between the thumb

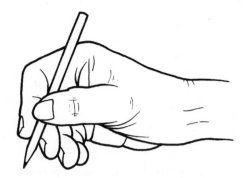

Figure 5.6   Writing with a pencil illustrates the fine controlled action that the lumbrical muscles are able to exert.

and index finger and print a large letter on a piece of paper. Notice the movements of the index finger joints. During the downstroke the IP joints flex and the MCP joint extends. At the upstroke flexion occurs at the MCP joint and the IP joints extend, i.e. you have flexed a straight finger – the action of the lumbricals (Fig. 5.6). The little finger has an additional small flexor, the flexor digiti minimi, found in the hypothenar eminence.

Such delicate movements need fine variations in tension in the extensor expansion, and the lumbricals have a perfect origin and insertion to modulate the basic movements of flexion and extension. They originate from the flexor digitorum profundus and insert into the extensor expansion.

Deviation either towards the ulnar or radial side is also possible in the MCP joints. The **interossei** are perfectly situated to produce these movements of radial or ulnar deviation (abduction/adduction movements in the classical terminology). The little finger, however, needs a special ulnar deviator. This is the **abductor digiti minimi** of the hypothenar group of muscles. The little finger metacarpal can also rotate in its long axis, so deepening the cup of the palm. This is produced by the **opponens digiti minimi** found in the hypothenar muscle group. Further insight into finger movements can be gained only after we have studied the movements of the thumb.

The deep extensors of the hand

The **deep group** of muscles on the back of the forearm arise from the posterior surfaces of the forearm bones and the interosseous membrane. (Compare these

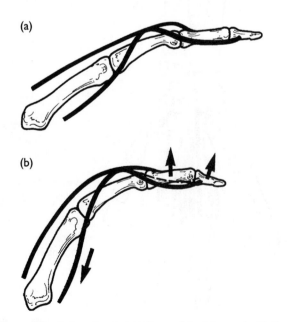

Figure 5.5   Pull on the straight fibres of the interossei with the finger positioned as shown in (a) flexes the MCP joint but extends the IP joints (b).

again with the deep group on the front of the forearm in Figure 4.14.) One of these muscles, the **extensor indicis**, has already been studied since it belongs functionally with all the other extensors of the fingers. Three of the other deep muscles act on the **thumb**. There are both long and short extensor muscles for the thumb, the **extensor pollicis longus** and **brevis** (Fig. 5.7). The long extensor of the thumb arises from the posterior surface of the ulna and the interosseous membrane. It passes over the distal end of the radius and through an osseofascial compartment. Here it lies in contact with the lower end of the radius. If you look at this region on a radius you will notice a small bony tubercle. The extensor pollicis longus runs around this tubercle, changing direction as it does. The insertion of extensor pollicis longus is into the distal phalanx of the thumb. The extensor pollicis brevis arises from the radius and interosseous membrane and passes through an osseofascial tunnel to its insertion at the base of the proximal phalanx of the thumb. The longus extends both IP and MCP joints of the thumb but the brevis extends only the MCP joint. Do not forget, however, the plane in which thumb movements take place (turn back to Figures 3.15 and 3.16). Both muscles are supplied by the posterior interosseous branch of the radial nerve.

The third muscle in the group of thumb muscles we are studying is the **abductor pollicis longus**. It arises from both forearm bones and interosseous membrane and accompanies the short extensor of the thumb through an osseofascial tunnel (Fig. 5.8). It is inserted into the base of the thumb metacarpal. Its action is therefore to abduct the metacarpal of the thumb. It is also supplied by the posterior interosseous branch of the radial nerve. If you are a fairly thin person, abducting and extending your thumb will make each of these three thumb tendons stand out. The concavity produced (see Fig. 5.8) is called the anatomical 'snuff box'. It was into this area (when it was fashionable) that a pinch of snuff could usefully be placed before sniffing it into the nose. The **scaphoid bone** can be palpated in the floor of the anatomical snuff box. This is an important point to remember because tenderness here after a wrist injury will almost certainly mean a fracture of this bone. These fractures are seen fairly frequently in any large emergency department. This is now a good time to review the movements of the thumb since all the muscles that control it have been studied.

The thumb metacarpal is very mobile and so its movements have to be studied carefully. The MCP joint can perform all the movements that are seen in the other MCP joints, that is, flexion, extension, abduction, and adduction. The IP joint, however, allows only flexion and extension.

The thumb metacarpal moves on the trapezium in a special way. The joint between the two bones is called a 'saddle joint' and it allows a rotational movement of the thumb metacarpal. It travels up, over and down the saddle-shaped surface of the trapezium, while turning through a gentle arc at the same time. The metacarpal may also be **adducted towards** the palm by the **adductor pollicis** or **abducted away** from the palm by the **abductor pollicis longus**. The rotation about the long axis of the thumb metacarpal occurs through the action of the **opponens pollicis**. This latter movement swings the shaft of the thumb metacarpal around so that the pulp of the thumb now faces the

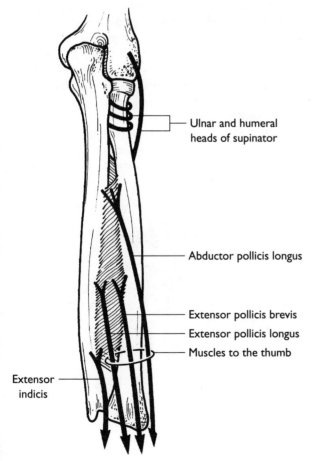

Ulnar and humeral heads of supinator

Abductor pollicis longus

Extensor pollicis brevis

Extensor pollicis longus

Muscles to the thumb

Extensor indicis

Figure 5.7 The deep group of extensor muscles on the back of the forearm.

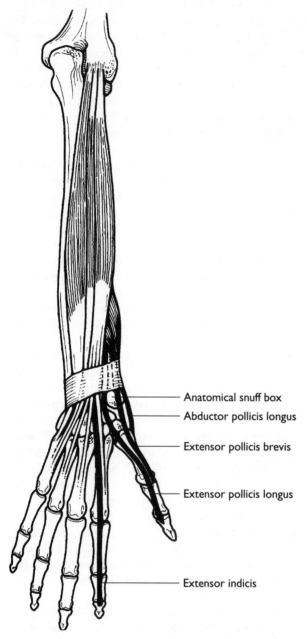

Anatomical snuff box

Abductor pollicis longus

Extensor pollicis brevis

Extensor pollicis longus

Extensor indicis

Figure 5.8   The tendons that define the anatomical snuff box and the extensor indicis tendon.

in an inability to perform the precision grip of thumb–finger opposition. This is a tremendous disability. Think for a moment how many times during the day this pad-to-pad pinch grip is used and how essential it is to normal everyday life. Loss of movement of the thumb is serious and is counted as 40% disability as far as the hand is concerned.

The MCP joint of the thumb is **flexed** by both the flexor pollicis longus and brevis. It is **extended** by the extensor pollicis longus and brevis. Like the other MCP joints it can deviate towards the ulnar or radial side. Radial deviation (**abduction**) is produced by the abductor pollicis brevis, and ulnar deviation (**adduction**) by the first palmar interosseous muscle and by the adductor pollicis. Hold your thumb metacarpal firmly; notice that the amount of deviation (abduction and adduction) that is possible in the thumb MCP joint is much less than that in the fingers. Movement in the thumb takes place at the synovial joint at the base of the metacarpal. The IP joint movement in the thumb is limited to flexion and extension. Flexion is produced by the flexor pollicis longus and extension by the extensor pollicis longus. Armed with the basic background knowledge of the function of the fingers and thumb outlined in this book you should now be able sensibly to assess injury or disease in the hand and fingers.

The last of the deep muscles to be studied on the back of the forearm is the **supinator** (Fig. 5.9). The supinator arises from stable bones, the ulna and

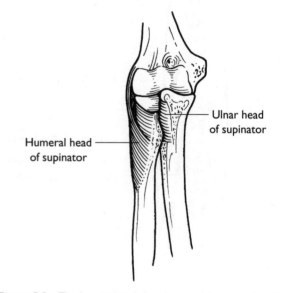

Ulnar head
of supinator

Humeral head
of supinator

pulp of the other fingertips. This is used to perform a precision type of grip. If you pinch the thumb to one or other of your fingers you will find that it is really a combined movement of **abduction** and **opposition** of the thumb metacarpal. The metacarpal may be returned to the side of the hand by the adductor pollicis. Loss of these important thumb metacarpal movements following either nerve or muscle injury results

Figure 5.9   The humeral and ulnar heads of the supinator muscle insert into the shaft of the radius.

humerus in this case, and inserts into the mobile radius. (Remember this is true of all supinators and pronators.) In fact the supinator arises as two heads from both the ulna and the lateral epicondylar region of the humerus. The ulnar head arises from the ulna just below the radial notch. It sweeps around from the back of the radius to insert into the anterior aspect of the radius. Some fibres of the supinator arise from the humerus in the region of the lateral epicondyle.

These run to the lateral aspect of the proximal third of the radius, so forming a humeral head. The muscle is supplied by the deep branch of the radial nerve.

The supinator, as its name implies, supinates the forearm. The other great supinating muscle that we studied previously is the biceps muscle. But the biceps cannot supinate while the arm is straight. The supinator, however, is capable of supination in any position of the arm.

Neurovascular Structures in the Arm, Hand and Digits

Trace now the neurovascular structures as they weave through the forearm into the hand and digits. You must learn the nerves carefully since injury to one or other of these is always serious. Arteries and veins in the forearm and hand can often be lacerated without fear of impairment of the vascular supply since, on the whole, there is a rich collateral network of vessels. First, let us review the neurovascular pattern in front of the elbow. The large nerves and vessels of the upper limb in this region were last seen lying in an intermuscular cleft called the **cubital fossa**. Look at this fossa a little more closely, paying particular attention to the pattern of neurovascular structures (Fig. 6.1). The intermuscular cleft is bounded by

Brachioradialis

Humeral head of supinator

Ulnar head of supinator

Brachialis

Biceps tendon

Superficial muscles cut

Pronator teres

Figure 6.1 The muscles that define and surround the cubital fossa.

the **pronator teres** on the ulnar side and the **brachioradialis** on the radial side. These two muscles arising from medial and lateral epicondylar regions, respectively, converge, thus giving the cubital fossa a triangular appearance. There is of course no 'base' to the triangle: this is merely an imaginary line joining the two epicondyles. When the pronator teres and brachioradialis are retracted, two muscles can be seen deeply placed in the 'floor' of the fossa. The insertion of the supinator conceals the upper part of the radius, and the insertion of the brachialis into the ulna produces a fleshy floor to the fossa. The capsule of the elbow joint is therefore for the most part concealed. The tendon of the biceps muscle dips into the cubital fossa to insert into the radius. This is a good landmark which can always be palpated during any procedure in this region. The bicipital aponeurosis spreads over the pronator teres, blending with the deep fascia on the ulnar side of the forearm.

The **brachial artery** with the **median nerve** on its *medial* side enters the fossa to the *medial* side of the biceps tendon. Palpate the biceps tendon at your elbow. The brachial artery may be felt pulsating on its medial side. This relationship is useful to remember since it is over this part of the brachial artery that stethoscope is placed when taking blood pressure (Fig. 6.2). The brachial artery divides into **radial** and **ulnar arteries**. The radial artery leaves the fossa through its apex and the ulnar artery leaves with the median nerve by passing deep to the pronator teres.

The **radial nerve** is apparent only if the brachioradialis is strongly retracted (Fig. 6.2). It will be seen lying on the surface of the supinator muscle. Here it divides into its two terminal branches. The **superficial**

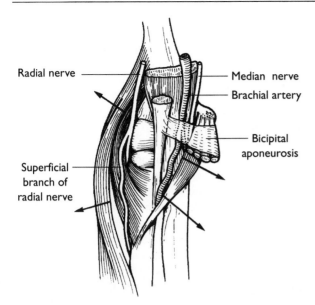

Figure 6.2   Brachialis and pronator teres have been retracted to reveal the neurovascular structures in the cubital fossa.

branch leaves the fossa by travelling deep to the brachioradialis and the **deep branch** is soon lost from view since it dips between the two heads of the supinator to reach the back of the forearm.

The **ulnar nerve** is not seen at the front of the elbow. It was traced previously to its position behind the medial epicondyle of the humerus. It can be palpated in this position. Be sure that you understand the basic positions of the neurovascular structures in the cubital fossa before proceeding to study their courses through the forearm and hand. Study the nerves first.

The **median nerve** leaves the medial side of the brachial artery by passing deep to the pronator teres. To follow its course further the muscles that form the 'roof' of the forearm have to be removed (pronator teres, flexor carpi radialis, palmaris longus and flexor carpi ulnaris); see Figure 6.3. The nerve can now be seen passing under the bridge of origin of the flexor digitorum superficialis. It travels down the forearm, 'stuck' to the deep surface of that muscle by a little areolar tissue. At the wrist the nerve emerges on the radial side of the superficialis tendons and passes with them through the osseofascial tunnel under the flexor retinaculum. (Since it does not move like the tendons it does not require a synovial sheath.) Before leaving the wrist it lies to the ulnar side of the flexor carpi radialis and is also often covered by the palmaris longus tendon. However, deep lacerations in this

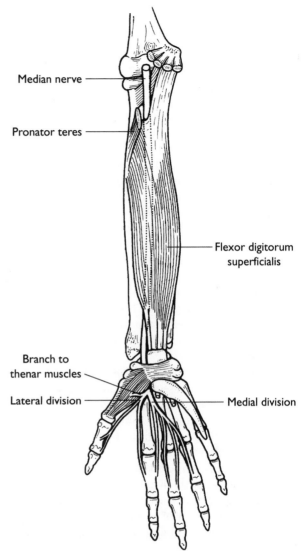

Figure 6.3   The median nerve and its relationship to the flexor digitorum superficialis in the forearm.

region do sometimes cut through the nerve. In the forearm the nerve gives branches to the roof muscles, i.e. pronator teres, flexor carpi radialis and palmaris longus. However, it does *not* supply the flexor carpi ulnaris. It also supplies the flexor digitorum superficialis. As the nerve passes under the bridge of the superficialis it gives off a branch called the **anterior interosseous nerve**. This supplies the deep muscles of the forearm, i.e. the flexor pollicis longus, the pronator teres and most of the flexor digitorum profundus. It gives a small cutaneous branch to the palmar skin. Once the median nerve has entered the palm after passing through the osseofascial tunnel, it divides into **lateral** and **medial** branches.

The **lateral** division gives a branch that supplies the thenar muscles. It then divides into three digital branches which carry sensations from the skin over the thumb and radial side of the index finger. It gives a branch to supply the first lumbrical muscle.

The **medial** division divides into two branches which head for the 2nd and 3rd interdigital clefts. They enter the fingers and are responsible for carrying sensation from the skin of the ulnar half of the index, middle and radial half of the ring fingers. The branches that travel on either side of thumb and fingers are called the **digital nerves**. Sensation is most sensitive over the pulps of the fingers and thumb. The digital branches of the median nerve not only supply palmar skin sensation but also carry sensory impulses from the skin of the nail beds on the dorsum of the thumb and fingers (Fig. 6.4). The area supplied by the median nerve is therefore the radial three and a half digits including the dorsal skin and nail beds at the tips of these digits.

The median nerve is in a protected position as it passes through the osseofascial tunnel at the wrist, and just proximal to this it is often covered by the tendon of palmaris longus. Sometimes, however, the nerve becomes compressed within the osseofascial tunnel. This condition often occurs in women. There are many causes; amongst them are swelling of the synovial sheaths of the flexor tendons in rheumatoid arthritis or generalized retention of fluid in the body tissues. The condition of nerve compression is called the **carpal tunnel syndrome**. Occasionally, the nerve

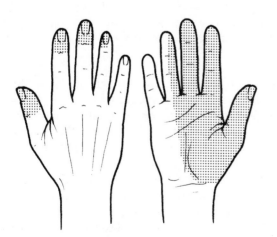

Figure 6.4 The cutaneous distribution of the median nerve on the front and back of the hand.

is lacerated at the wrist in accidents, such as, for example, where the hand is forced through a glass window or during other industrial accidents. Whichever way the median nerve is damaged at the wrist, loss of function in the hand follows the same pattern. There is a loss of **sensation** and a loss of **muscular action**. Sensation is lost over a very important area of the hand (Fig. 6.4). To be able to pick up objects and feel their shape, sensation is essential, especially over the pulps of the thumb and index and middle fingers. In median nerve interruption, sensation is lost over the thumb, index and middle fingers and half the ring finger on their palmar surface. The nail beds are also numb. If the laceration is a little above the wrist the cutaneous nerve to the palm may also be damaged, producing numbness over the radial half of the palm. The loss of nerve supply to the **thenar muscles** also causes deformity. The thenar eminence loses its fullness and appears flat. The thumb also tends to lie flat, in the same plane as the rest of the fingers. The most important muscle loss is the opponens pollicis so that opposition of the thumb to a finger is impossible. The patient finds difficulty in picking things up and holding them. He or she can manage a 'trick' movement in an attempt to oppose the thumb by using the flexor pollicis longus, but this is very awkward. Loss of the lateral two lumbrical muscle actions does not seem to produce deformity.

The **ulnar nerve** approaches the forearm from behind the medial epicondyle (Fig. 6.5). It passes between the two heads of origin of the flexor carpi ulnaris, and in this way reaches the deep surface of the roof muscles. It travels down the forearm deep to the flexor carpi ulnaris, along the edge of the flexor digitorum superficialis. Notice that the **superficialis** holds a key muscular relationship to the **median** and **ulnar** nerves. At the wrist the ulnar nerve becomes superficial at the radial side of the flexor carpi ulnaris tendon and here it passes on to the *surface* of the flexor retinaculum. It does *not*, therefore, pass into the palm through the osseofascial carpal tunnel like the median nerve. You will see, however, that it is protected on the surface of the retinaculum by a fibrous sheet and so is not completely exposed. While passing over the retinaculum it lies at the side of the pisiform bone and this is a good way to locate its position in the wrist. In the region of the wrist it gives, like the median nerve, a cutaneous branch to the palm. However, unlike the median nerve, it also gives a **dorsal cutaneous branch** which arises well above the wrist

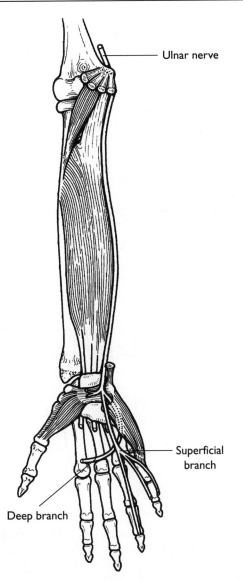

Figure 6.5 The ulnar nerve and its relationship to the edge of the flexor digitorum superficialis where it lies deep to flexor carpi ulnaris.

then dips into the palm between the flexor digiti minimi brevis and the abductor digiti minimi, supplying all three hypothenar muscles on the way. In the palm it passes over the palmar surface of the metacarpals deep to the long tendons. It supplies all the deep muscles in the palm, i.e. all the interosseous muscles, the adductor pollicis and the medial two lumbricals.

The ulnar nerve can be injured during lacerations at the wrist or following injuries or deformities of the elbow. Following a laceration at the wrist, there will be loss of sensation and of muscular action. There is anaesthesia of the palmar surfaces of the little finger and half the ring finger, and loss of sensation on the dorsum of these fingers including the region of the nail bed (Fig. 6.6). The hypothenar muscles will be paralysed and will waste. To determine this lack of hypothenar power easily, one can test the action of the abductor digiti minimi. Ask the patient to abduct the little finger and they will be unable to perform this movement. The interossei are also wasted in an ulnar nerve lesion, which is usually obvious from the sunken appearance of the interosseous spaces on the back of the hand. The first web is thin and wasted due to degeneration of the adductor pollicis and the first dorsal interosseous muscle. Because the medial two lumbricals are paralysed the balance between flexors and extensors of the ring and little fingers is lost. This results in a peculiar 'claw type' of deformity of these fingers called claw hand (Fig. 6.7). If the ulnar nerve is interrupted at the elbow, the flexor carpi ulnaris is also paralysed.

The **radial nerve** was last seen in front of the elbow by retracting the brachioradialis muscle. Here it lies

and carries sensation from the ulnar side of the dorsum of the hand and fingers. While in the forearm it supplies the **flexor carpi ulnaris** and part of the **flexor digitorum profundus.**

As the nerve passes the pisiform bone it divides into a **superficial** and a **deep branch** (Fig. 6.5). The **superficial branch** supplies only one muscle, the small palmaris brevis. Its main function is to carry cutaneous sensation from the medial one and a half digits, on their palmar surfaces and the skin of the nail beds. The deep branch skirts the hook of the hamate and

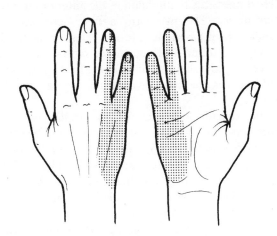

Figure 6.6 The cutaneous distribution of the ulnar nerve on the front and back of the hand.

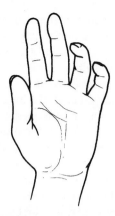

Figure 6.7　Loss of function of the medial two lumbricals in an ulnar nerve lesion leads to a loss of balance between the flexors and extensors of the ring and little finger. The result is a deformity called claw hand.

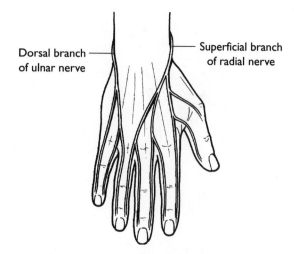

Dorsal branch of ulnar nerve　　Superficial branch of radial nerve

Figure 6.8　The superficial branch of the radial nerve runs over the anatomical snuff box on to the back of the hand.

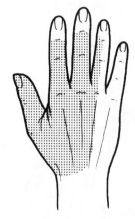

Figure 6.9　The cutaneous distribution of the superficial branch of the radial nerve on the back of the hand.

on the supinator muscle and here also it divides into **superficial** and **deep branches** (Fig. 6.2). The deep branch continues to the back of the forearm by passing between the two heads of the supinator muscle. It is destined to supply *all* the extensor musculature of the forearm. With this must be included a supply to the brachioradialis, which was originally an extensor muscle. On arrival at the back of the forearm this deep branch is renamed the **posterior interosseous nerve**. Here it joins an artery of similar name and the neurovascular bundle passes down deep to the extensor digitorum, that is between the superficial and deep layers of the extensor musculature. At about the middle of the forearm, the nerve dips deeply to gain the posterior aspect of the interosseous membrane. Here it meets the termination of the **anterior interosseous artery**. The two form a new neurovascular bundle which passes deep to the extensor digitorum through its tunnel in the extensor retinaculum. The nerve ends in a slight swelling at the back of the wrist and supplies the wrist joint with several articular twigs.

The **superficial branch** of the radial nerve is cutaneous. It passes down in company with the radial artery, deep to the brachioradialis, to reach the lower end of the radius. It winds around to the back of the forearm, passing over the anatomical snuffbox as it does so (Fig. 6.8). It is responsible for sensation on the back of the hand, thumb and lateral two and a half fingers (Fig. 6.9) (like the median nerve on the palmar aspect). The supply stops short of the nail beds, which are supplied by the median nerve. The ulnar one and

a half digits are supplied by a dorsal branch of the ulnar nerve.

We have seen earlier how the radial nerve can be damaged in the axilla, from the pressure of a crutch bearing the weight of the body, for example, or following fracture of the humeral shaft. Fractures or dislocations of the head of the radius can also damage the posterior interosseous branch supplying the extensor muscles of the forearm. Damage to the radial nerve results in '**wrist drop**' (Fig. 6.10). Damage to the posterior interosseous nerve leaves the extensor carpi radialis intact though, since it is supplied by the radial nerve before it divides. Wrist drop leaves the flexor muscles too slack to grip firmly. Anaesthesia in a radial nerve lesion is usually most intense between the

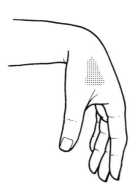

Figure 6.10 Damage to the radial nerve results in wrist drop and an area of anaesthesia between the thumb and 1st metacarpal.

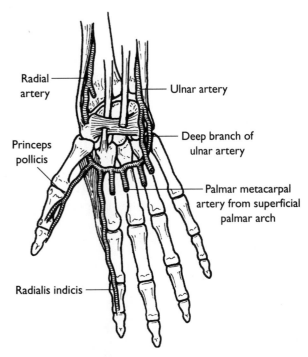

Figure 6.11 Branches of the radial and ulnar arteries in the hand.

thumb and first metacarpal on the back of the hand (Fig. 6.10).

All that remains now is to study the **radial artery** and **ulnar artery** and then the pattern of venous drainage of the upper limb. The vascular pattern, especially in the palm of the hand, is variable. The collateral circulations of the forearm and hand are very free. Even a large artery like the radial artery may be divided without impairment of the circulation in the hand. It is only in certain instances that there is a complete 'cut off' in blood supply to the hand, such as a consequence of severe swelling of the elbow region following fracture of the lower humerus in a child. You should, therefore, concentrate on learning the nerve supply of the upper limb, since nerves in this region are frequently injured during accidents. Both their course and position need to be learned. However, it is useful to be aware of the usual pattern of the distal ends of the radial and ulnar arteries in the hand.

The **radial artery** is one of the terminal branches of the brachial artery. It leaves the cubital fossa at its apex and passes downwards along the edge of the superficial 'roof' muscles in company with the superficial branch of the radial nerve (Figs 6.11 and 6.12). The two are hidden from view by the overlapping brachioradialis muscle. This muscle, originally an extensor, can clearly be seen arising from the lateral epicondylar region and passing down to its insertion into the lower part of the shaft of the radius. As the radial artery approaches the wrist it becomes more exposed between the tendons of the brachioradialis and flexor carpi radialis. Here it can be felt pulsating in the living limb and is commonly used for feeling

the radial pulse in this position. While in the forearm, the radial artery supplies the forearm muscles and also helps to supply the elbow and wrist joints with blood.

The artery passes around the lower end of the radius and crosses the anatomical snuffbox deep to the tendons. In this way it reaches the first intermetacarpal cleft. Here it dips between the two heads of the first dorsal interosseous muscle (Fig. 6.11). At this point it gives off a branch to the index finger called the radialis indicis and a branch to the thumb, the princeps pollicis. Having done this the artery continues between the two heads of the adductor pollicis to arrive in the intermediate compartment of the palm on a plane that is *deep* to all the long tendons passing through. Here, on the surface of the metacarpals, it forms the **deep palmar arch** by anastomosing on the ulnar side of the palm with the deep branch of the ulnar artery. Three palmar metacarpal arteries arise from the deep arch. They supply blood to the metacarpals and deep muscles of the palm, and help to reinforce the blood supply of the fingers.

The **ulnar artery** is the other terminal branch of the brachial artery. It leaves the cubital fossa by passing deep to the pronator teres (Fig. 6.11). It passes,

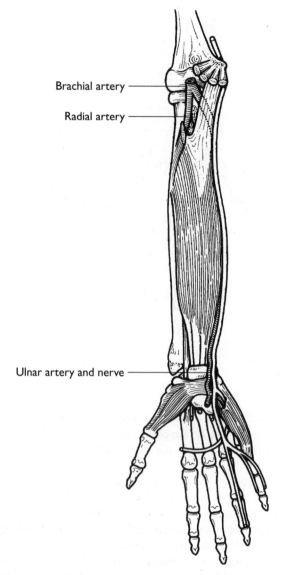

Figure 6.12   The ulnar artery in company with the ulnar nerve at the wrist.

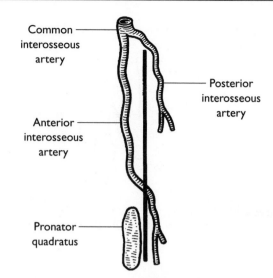

Figure 6.13   The dark line represents the interosseous membrane. The common interosseous artery splits and the anterior interosseous artery first travels in front of the membrane but then passes through it, behind pronator quadratus, before anastomosing on the back of the hand with the posterior interosseous artery.

The **posterior interosseous artery** pierces the membrane and reaches the posterior aspect of the forearm to nourish muscles there. The **anterior interosseous artery** descends in company with the anterior interosseous branch of the median nerve as far as the pronator quadratus; it then also pierces the interosseous membrane to reach the back of the forearm. Here, at its termination, it joins the termination of the posterior interosseous nerve. The artery helps in the supply of a vascular network on the back of the wrist and hand.

The main part of the ulnar artery meets the ulnar nerve at the ulnar side of the flexor digitorum superficialis (Fig. 6.12). Both artery and nerve pass on to the surface of the flexor retinaculum and both divide into superficial and deep branches. The **deep branches** of both nerve and artery curve around the hook of the hamate and sink between the hypothenar muscles to gain the deep plane of the palm. The deep branch of the artery ends by anastomosing with the termination of the radial artery to form the deep palmar arch.

The superficial branch of the artery is the continuation that passes onwards over the retinaculum. It then arches laterally on a superficial plane in the palm as the **superficial palmar arch** (Fig. 6.14). The arch is usually completed by anastomosis with a small

with the median nerve, beneath the origin of the flexor digitorum superficialis. However, unlike the nerve which passes straight down the forearm (Fig. 6.3), the ulnar artery veers to the ulnar side of the deep surface of the superficialis, so reaching its namesake, the ulnar nerve (Figs 6.5 and 6.12). While in the forearm the artery supplies blood to the forearm muscles and also supplies blood as a vascular network around the elbow joint. Its main branch is the **common interosseous artery** (Fig. 6.13). The artery divides at the upper part of the interosseous membrane.

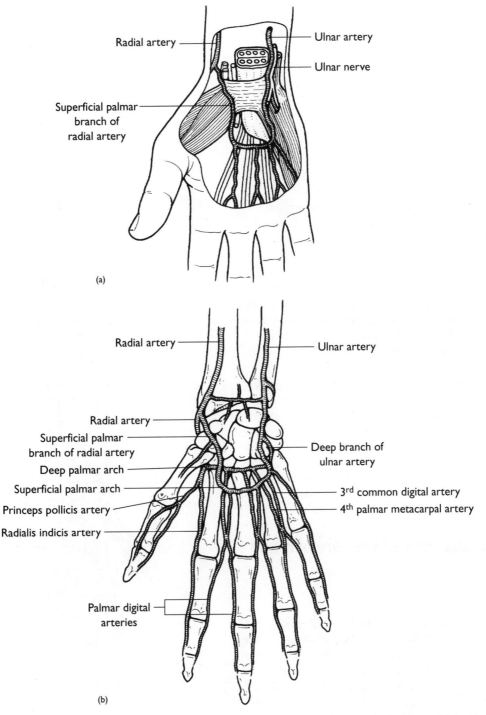

Figure 6.14 (a) The superficial palmar arch: the 5th digital artery usually remains undivided. (b) Both superficial and deep palmar arches are illustrated with the palmar metacarpal and digital arteries and the princeps pollicis.

branch of the radial artery. The arch lies not only more superficial to the deep arch but also more distal. It is usually at the level of the proximal palmar crease. From the convexity of the arch, arteries pass to the digits. The pattern is variable, but usually the fifth digital artery remains undivided and travels along the ulnar side of the little finger in company with the digital nerve. The others arise as common digital arteries, which each divide into two digital arteries at an interdigital cleft. Each digital artery accompanies its corresponding nerve and at the end of the digit forms a free capillary network in the pulp of the digit and nail bed.

Each of the main arteries of the upper limb is accompanied by a vein, or pair of veins. A network of superficial veins courses over the back of the hand and runs either laterally, to form the **cephalic vein**, or more medially to form the **basilic vein** (Fig. 6.15). The cephalic vein begins superficial to the styloid process of the radius. It comes to lie in a groove along the lateral border of the biceps muscle. It then goes on to pierce deep fascia and then clavipectoral fascia in the groove between deltoid and pectoralis major, and enters the **axillary vein**. The basilic vein runs on the medial aspect of the forearm, crosses the elbow and pierces the deep fascia of the upper arm. From here it runs in the posterior axillary fold to join the axillary vein high in the axilla. The cephalic and basilic veins are usually joined obliquely across the cubital fossa by a **median cubital vein**. Veins on the back of the hand and around the cubital fossa are often used for venepuncture and transfusion.

Applied anatomy of the forearm and hand

Fractures of bones

Fractures of the lower end of the humerus just above the epicondyles illustrate an important point. This kind of fracture usually occurs in children and is often fairly easily reduced. However, there is always a certain amount of swelling of the tissues after any injury and supracondylar fracture of the humerus is no exception. The arm is placed in a sling after reduction and, if the elbow is bent to a right angle, the swelling in the cubital fossa region will sometimes be enough to occlude the flow of blood through the brachial artery. All such children, therefore, are carefully followed over the first 24 hours or so, with repeated

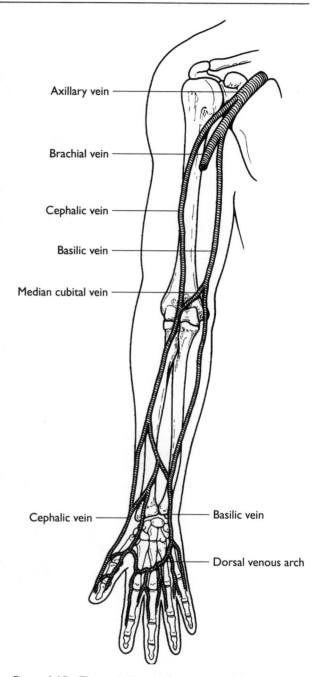

Axillary vein

Brachial vein

Cephalic vein

Basilic vein

Median cubital vein

Cephalic vein — — Basilic vein

— Dorsal venous arch

Figure 6.15 The cephalic vein forms superficial to the radial styloid. The basilic vein forms on the medial side of the back of the wrist. Both eventually join the axillary vein in the axilla.

examinations to determine whether the radial pulse is still palpable. If the pulse cannot be felt at any time the elbow must be straightened a little.

The radius is a bone that is fractured relatively frequently. There are certain sites at which the bone fractures most commonly (Fig. 6.16). The neck or head of the radius may be fractured. Such a break often heals well unless the head has been dislocated or the articular surface badly shattered. Fractures of the shaft of the radius are often accompanied by fractures of the ulna. In children, such breaks often do not completely fracture through the bone. The resulting incomplete break is called a 'greenstick type' of fracture. In adults fractures tend to be complete and accurate replacement of the bone ends is essential to prevent severe limitation of movement and function. Pronation and supination are often affected if the reduction has been inaccurate. Probably the most frequently seen fracture is in the lower one inch of the radius. This is often associated with fracture of the styloid process of the ulna, and is named after the Irish physician who first described it: a Colles' fracture. It occurs often in the elderly who fall on an outstretched hand. The broken distal end of the radius is impacted into the proximal part of the bone and is also tilted dorsally (Fig. 6.17). It is also deviated to the radial side (Fig. 6.18). All this has to be reduced when the bones are set. In young adults who have this type of fracture before growth of their bones is completed, the bone fractures across the lower growth plate of the radius. This is a so-called fractured radial epiphysis.

In the wrist, the bone most frequently fractured is the **scaphoid**. This usually fractures across its waist (Fig. 6.19). It is a common fracture of young adults.

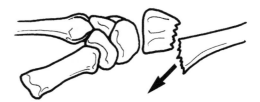

Figure 6.17 A Colles' fracture (in the lower one inch of the radius). The distal end of the bone is tilted dorsally and impacted into the proximal end of the shaft.

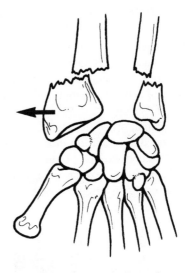

Figure 6.18 Here the distal end of the fractured radius is shown displaced to the radial side of the wrist.

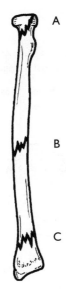

Figure 6.16 Fractures of the radius occur either at its head or neck (A), along the shaft (B) or in the lower one inch (C).

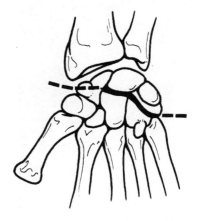

Figure 6.19 The scaphoid lies in the line of the midcarpal joint between the two rows of carpal bones.

Remember the surface anatomy of the scaphoid. It may be palpated deeply in the 'anatomical snuffbox', especially when the wrist is gently adducted. Tenderness in this region following injury should never be taken lightly. The scaphoid lies across the line of the midcarpal joint, between the two rows of carpal bones. In forced movement across this line the scaphoid is liable to crack (Fig. 6.20). Such a break takes a long time to heal. Occasionally, the blood supply to the proximal fragment is cut off by the fracture and the fragment dies.

Sprains, ruptured tendons and muscle insertions

Occasionally a tendon ruptures without being cut. For example, the tendon of extensor pollicis longus can sometimes rupture if it has been allowed to rub over the sharp edge of a badly treated Colles' fracture. A good example of tearing of a muscle at its attachment is seen in the condition of 'tennis elbow'. This condition is probably due to tearing of a few fibres at the origin of the common extensor tendon at the lateral epicondylar region during exercise. Activities that put tension on this common origin cause great pain.

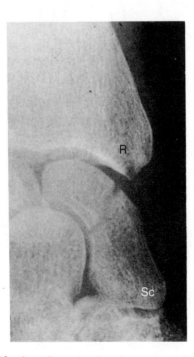

Figure 6.20 A radiograph of a fractured scaphoid. R, the styloid process of the radius; Sc, scaphoid bone.

Infections

Pus from infection of the hand can accumulate in either the **deep** or **superficial palmar spaces**, or in the **thenar space**. These are not real 'spaces' as such but areas limited by fascial boundaries which prevent the spread of pus from one to the other (Fig. 6.21). Deep infection of the palm can be caused by perforating injuries. In the superficial space of the mid-palm, pus may easily be drained with a surgical incision. However, care must be exercised in drainage of the deep and thenar 'spaces' to avoid injury to tendons, nerves and vessels. Apart from the loose areolar tissue in the so-called 'spaces' of the palm, infections may also be seen in the **synovial sheaths** of the tendons. Infection of the fingers may involve the sheaths of the tendons as they run along the osseofascial tunnel of the digit. Generally speaking they will be localized for some time to the finger except in the case of the little finger or thumb. The digital sheath of the little finger is continuous with the common synovial sheath and so infection here may quickly pass into the common sheath. Similarly, the thumb tendon sheath will spread along the sheath of the flexor pollicis longus as far as the wrist. Infections of the sheaths are called tenosynovitis, and pus formed in them must be carefully drained. If adequate treatment is not given, infection can eventually interfere with the blood supply of the tendons themselves and even cause rupture of the sheath. Surgical incisions in the hand and fingers need to be carefully placed so that no neurovascular

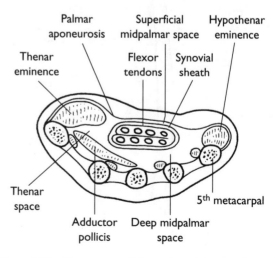

Figure 6.21 The spaces of the palm of the hand are sites where infection is common.

structures are damaged, and also with consideration for a scar that will heal quickly. A good example of this is a severe infection in the pulp of the finger which should be incised at the sides of the terminal phalanx and not opened through the fingertip since a scar on the fingertip is always inconvenient and will make future use of the finger difficult.

Summary and Revision of the Upper Limb

First use Figures 7.1, 7.2, 7.3 and 7.4 to revise both the course of the major nerves and the nerve supply to each of the muscles of the upper limb. Next read through the brief summaries of each muscle in each region of the upper limb and remind yourself about the origins, insertions and actions of each one. **Do not try to learn origins and insertions in too much detail.** Try to understand them and visualize them, and you will retain sufficient detail to answer the questions set out next. Finally, to bring together what you have learned, go through the multiple choice questions at the end of this chapter. For each **stem**, any one of the

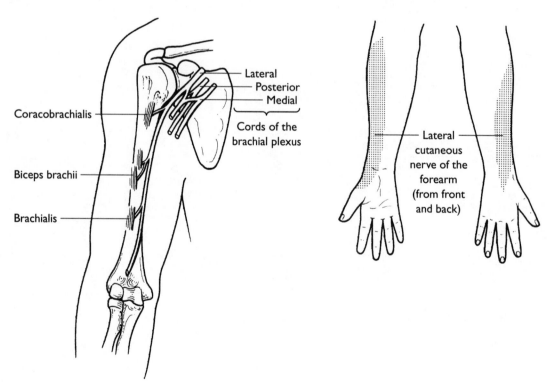

Figure 7.1 The course and distribution of the musculocutaneous nerve (after Hollinshead, WH (1982) *Anatomy for Surgeons*, 3rd edn. Philadelphia: Harper and Row). Note that the lateral cutaneous nerve of the forearm is a branch of the musculocutaneous nerve but that the medial cutaneous nerves of the arm and forearm arise directly from the medial cord of the brachial plexus in the axilla (look back to Figure 1.20).

five answers (A–E) may be either correct or incorrect. Many of the multiple choice questions are quite difficult. On your first attempt at these questions a score of around 50% correct would be very reasonable. We expect you to have to refer back to the text to improve your score. In so doing, of course, your understanding of upper limb anatomy will greatly improve.

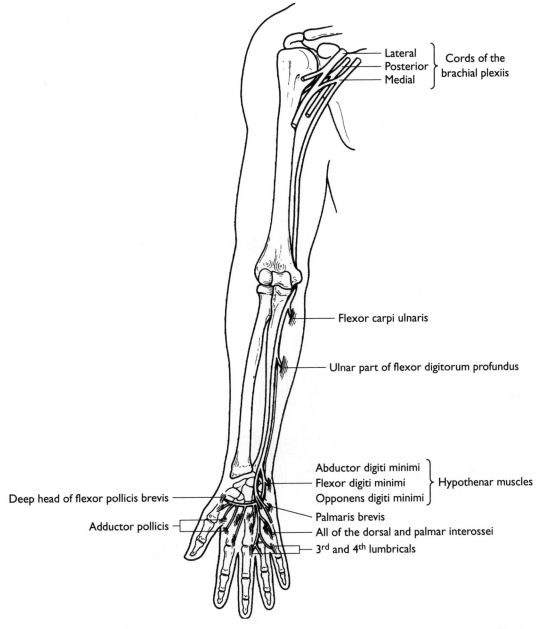

Figure 7.2 The course and distribution of the ulnar nerve in the arm, forearm and hand (after Hollinshead, WH (1982) *Anatomy for Surgeons*, 3rd edn. Philadelphia: Harper and Row). The cutaneous distribution of the ulnar nerve in the hand is illustrated in Figure 6.6.

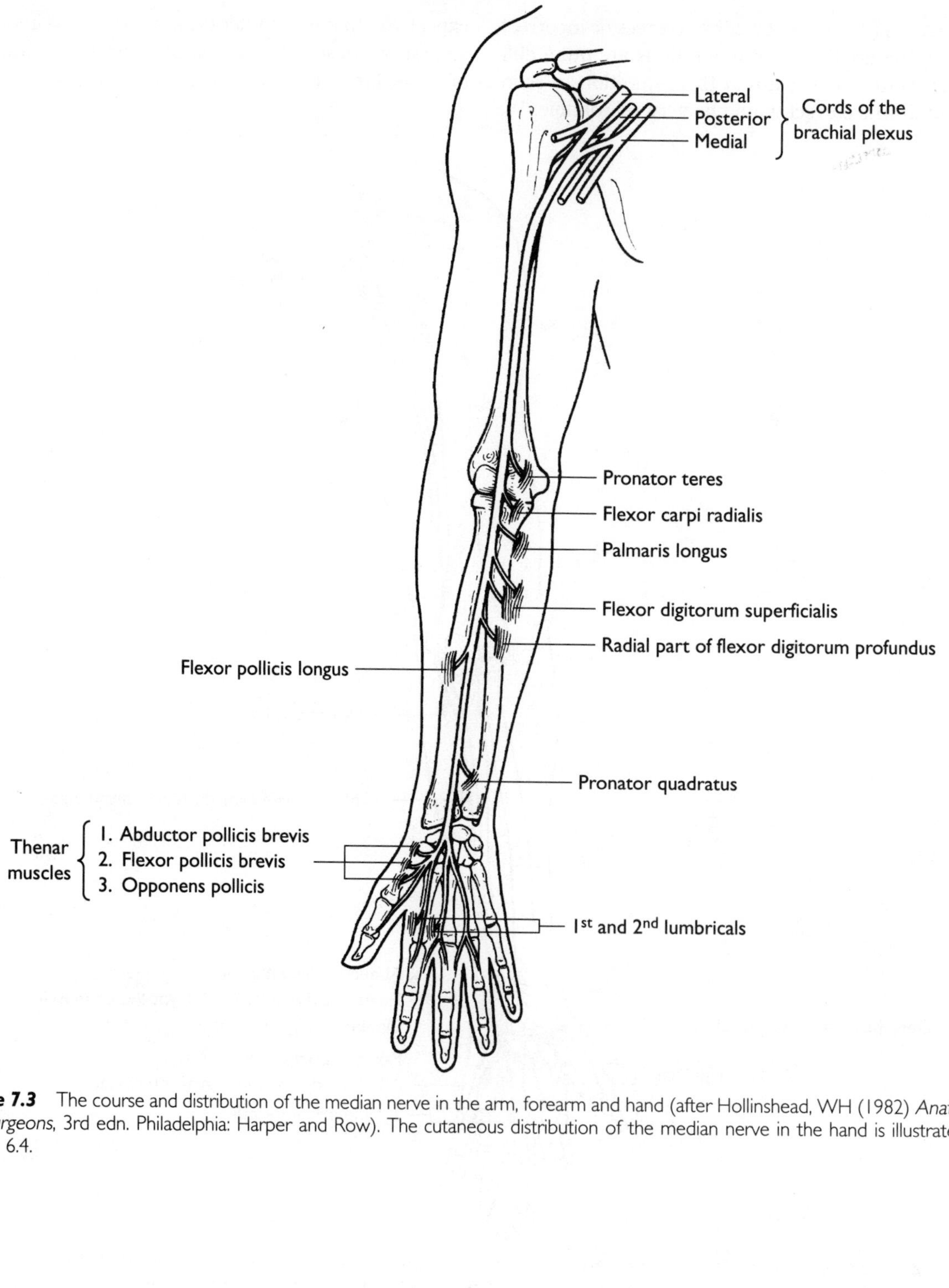

Lateral
Posterior
Medial
} Cords of the brachial plexus

Pronator teres

Flexor carpi radialis

Palmaris longus

Flexor digitorum superficialis

Radial part of flexor digitorum profundus

Flexor pollicis longus

Pronator quadratus

Thenar muscles {
1. Abductor pollicis brevis
2. Flexor pollicis brevis
3. Opponens pollicis

1st and 2nd lumbricals

Figure 7.3   The course and distribution of the median nerve in the arm, forearm and hand (after Hollinshead, WH (1982) *Anatomy for Surgeons*, 3rd edn. Philadelphia: Harper and Row). The cutaneous distribution of the median nerve in the hand is illustrated in Figure 6.4.

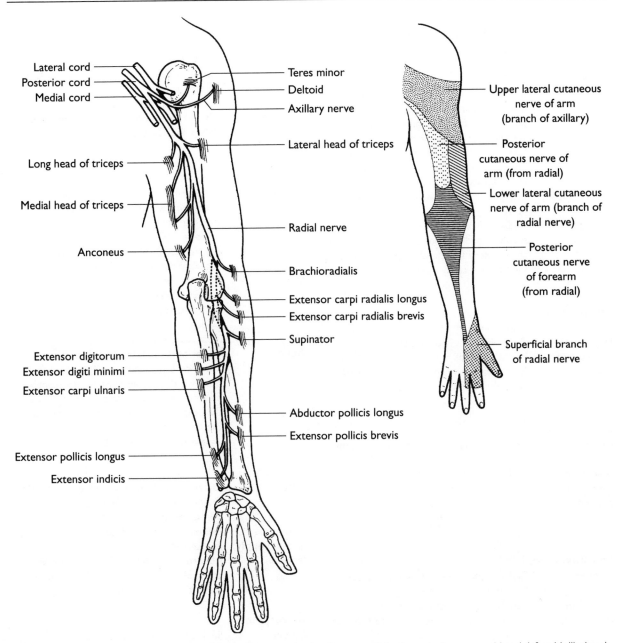

Figure 7.4 The course and distribution of the radial nerve (and axillary nerve) in the arm, forearm and hand (after Hollinshead, WH (1982) *Anatomy for Surgeons*, 3rd edn. Philadelphia: Harper and Row).

Muscles of the shoulder region

Pectoralis major
Origin: (i) Clavicular head: anterior surface of inner two-thirds of clavicle.
(ii) Sternocostal head: anterior surface of sternum and upper six ribs.

Insertion: Lateral crest of intertubercular groove. The lower fibres are inserted deep to the upper fibres.

Nerve supply: Lateral pectoral nerve and medial pectoral nerve.

Action: Adducts, flexes and medially rotates arm. If shoulder girdle is fixed, it can be used as an accessory muscle of respiration drawing the thoracic cavity upwards.

Pectoralis minor
Origin: Third, fourth and fifth ribs.
Insertion: Coracoid process of scapula.
Nerve supply: Medial pectoral.
Action: Either draws coracoid process forward and downwards or draws ribs upwards.

Subclavius
Origin: Junction of first costal cartilage and bony rib.
Insertion: Under surface of clavicle.
Nerve supply: Nerve to subclavius.
Action: Depresses lateral end of and stabilizes clavicle.

Serratus anterior
Origin: First to eighth ribs. Arises by digitations from the anterior ends.
Insertion: Vertebral border of the scapula.
Nerve supply: Nerve to serratus anterior (long thoracic nerve).
Action: Draws the scapula around the chest when pushing with the arm flexed.

Latissimus dorsi
Origin: (i) Vertebral spines, T7–S2.
(ii) Posterior part of iliac crest.
(iii) Slips from ninth to twelfth ribs.
Insertion: Intertubercular groove of the humerus.
Nerve supply: Thoracodorsal nerve.
Action: Adducts, medially rotates and extends the arm.

Levator scapulae
Origin: Tubercles of the transverse processes of the first and second cervical vertebrae. Posterior tubercles of the third and fourth cervical vertebrae.
Insertion: Vertebral border of scapula.
Nerve supply: C3 and C4 and dorsal scapular nerve C5.
Action: Raises the scapula and supports the upper limb.

Trapezius
Origin: (i) External occipital protuberance and inner third of superior nuchal line.
(ii) Ligamentum nuchae running from skull to spine of T12.
(iii) Vertebral spines from C7–T12 and supraspinous ligaments between them.
Insertion: (i) Upper border of spine of scapula.
(ii) Inner border of acromion.
(iii) Posterior border of outer third of clavicle.
Nerve supply: XI accessory nerve.
Action: Upper fibres pull the scapula and clavicle upwards. Lower fibres pull the scapula downwards. Whole muscle pulls scapula to midline. Trapezius is also used to rotate the scapula as when raising the arm above the head. The upper fibres support the weight of the upper limb.

Deltoid
Origin: Outer third of anterior surface of clavicle. Outer border of acromion and lower border of spine of scapula.
Insertion: Deltoid tuberosity of humerus.
Nerve supply: Axillary nerve.
Action: Abducts the humerus. The anterior fibres acting alone flex the arm. The posterior fibres extend the arm.

Supraspinatus
Origin: Supraspinous fossa of scapula.
Insertion: Greater tubercle of humerus (uppermost facet).
Nerve supply: Suprascapular.
Action: Abducts the humerus.

Infraspinatus
Origin: Infraspinous fossa of scapula.
Insertion: Greater tubercle of humerus (middle facet).
Nerve supply: Suprascapular nerve.
Action: Lateral rotator of the humerus, fixator of head of humerus.

Teres minor

Origin: Middle part of lateral border of scapula.

Insertion: Greater tubercle of humerus (lowest facet).

Nerve supply: Axillary nerve.

Action: Lateral rotator of the humerus, fixator of head.

Subscapularis

Origin: Subscapular fossa of scapula.

Insertion: Lesser tubercle of humerus.

Nerve supply: Subscapular nerves.

Action: Medial rotator of the humerus.

Teres major

Origin: Lower part of lateral border and inferior angle of scapula.

Insertion: Medial crest of intertubercular groove of humerus.

Nerve supply: Lower subscapular nerve.

Action: Adducts and medially rotates humerus.

Biceps brachii

Origin: Long head arises from the scapula just above the glenoid cavity. Short head arises from the tip of the coracoid process of the scapula.

Insertion: Posterior part of tuberosity of the radius and through the bicipital aponeurosis to the deep fascia over pronator teres.

Nerve supply: Musculocutaneous.

Action: Flexes the elbow and supinates the forearm.

Coracobrachialis

Origin: Tip of coracoid process of scapula.

Insertion: Middle of humeral shaft on medial side.

Nerve supply: Musculocutaneous nerve.

Action: Flexes and adducts the shoulder.

Brachialis

Origin: Lower two-thirds of anterior surface of humerus.

Insertion: Ulna, in front of coronoid process.

Nerve supply: Musculocutaneous nerve.

Action: Flexor of the elbow joint.

Triceps

Origin: Long head, from scapula below glenoid cavity. Lateral head, from ridge on humerus below greater tubercle. Medial head, from posterior surface of humerus below the spiral groove.

Insertion: Olecranon of ulna.

Nerve supply: Radial nerve.

Action: Extensor of the elbow joint.

Anconeus

Origin: Posterior aspect of lateral epicondyle of humerus.

Insertion: Upper quarter of posterior surface of ulna.

Nerve supply: Radial nerve.

Action: Weak extensor of elbow.

Flexors and pronators of the upper limb

Pronator teres

Origin: Medial epicondyle of the humerus.

Insertion: Lateral side of the shaft of the radius.

Nerve supply: Median nerve.

Action: Pronates the forearm. Flexes the elbow joint.

Pronator quadratus

Origin: Lower quarter of anterior surface of ulna.

Insertion: Anterior surface of radius.

Nerve supply: Anterior interosseous nerve (branch of median nerve).

Action: Pronates the forearm.

Brachioradialis

Origin: Upper two-thirds of lateral supracondylar ridge and lateral intermuscular septum.

Insertion: Just above styloid process of radius.

Nerve supply: Radial nerve.

Action: Flexes the elbow and rotates the forearm from either prone or supine position to mid-prone–supine position.

Flexor carpi radialis

Origin: Medial epicondyle of the humerus.

Insertion: Base of second and third metacarpals.

Nerve supply: Median nerve.

Action: Flexes the wrist.

Palmaris longus

Origin: Medial epicondyle of humerus.
Insertion: Palmar fascia.
Nerve supply: Median nerve.
Action: Flexes the wrist.

Flexor carpi ulnaris

Origin: From the medial epicondyle and the olecranon and upper two-thirds of posterior border of ulna.
Insertion: Pisiform bone.
Nerve supply: Ulnar nerve.
Action: Flexes and adducts the wrist.

Flexor digitorum superficialis

Origin: From the medial epicondyle, tubercle on the medial side of coronoid process of ulna and the anterior border of radius.
Insertion: Splits into four tendons at wrist. Inserted into sides of middle phalanges.
Nerve supply: Median nerve.
Action: Flexes proximal interphalangeal joints of the fingers.

Flexor digitorum profundus

Origin: Upper three-quarters of anterior and medial surface of ulna and interosseous membrane.
Insertion: Base of terminal phalanges.
Nerve supply: Anterior interosseous nerve (median nerve) and ulnar nerve (medial part).
Action: Flexes fingers and wrist.

Flexor pollicis longus

Origin: Anterior surface of radius and interosseous membrane.
Insertion: Terminal phalanx of thumb.
Nerve supply: Anterior interosseous nerve (median nerve).
Action: Flexes terminal phalanx of thumb.

Supinator and extensors of the upper limb

Supinator

Origin: Lateral epicondyle and ulna.
Insertion: Lateral aspect of radius.
Nerve supply: Posterior interosseous nerve.
Action: Supinates the forearm.

Extensor carpi radialis longus

Origin: Lower third of lateral epicondylar ridge and lateral intermuscular septum.
Insertion: Base of second metacarpal on dorsum of hand.
Nerve supply: Radial nerve.
Action: Extends and abducts the wrist.

Extensor carpi radialis brevis

Origin: Lateral epicondyle.
Insertion: Base of second and third metacarpals on dorsum of hand.
Nerve supply: Posterior interosseous nerve (radial nerve).
Action: Extends and abducts the wrist.

Extensor carpi ulnaris

Origin: Lateral epicondyle and part of posterior border of ulna.
Insertion: Base of fifth metacarpal on dorsum of hand.
Nerve supply: Posterior interosseous nerve (radial nerve).
Action: Extends and adducts the wrist,

Extensor digitorum

Origin: Lateral epicondyle
Insertion: Four tendons with slips to the proximal, middle and distal phalanges of each finger.
Nerve supply: Posterior interosseous nerve (radial nerve).
Action: Extends fingers and wrist. The main action is on the metacarpophalangeal joint of each finger.

Extensor indicis

Origin: Shaft of distal part of ulna.
Insertion: Tendon to index finger, joins extensor expansion.
Nerve supply: Posterior interosseous nerve.
Action: Extends index finger.

Extensor digiti minimi

Origin: Lateral epicondyle.
Insertion: To common extensor tendon of little finger.
Nerve supply: Posterior interosseous nerve (radial nerve).
Action: Extends little finger.

Abductor pollicis longus

Origin: Ulna, interosseous membrane, and radius.
Insertion: Base of thumb metacarpal.
Nerve supply: Posterior interosseous nerve.
Action: Abducts and also extends the thumb.

Extensor pollicis brevis

Origin: Radius and interosseous membrane.
Insertion: Base of proximal phalanx of thumb.
Nerve supply: Posterior interosseous nerve.
Action: Extends proximal phalanx of thumb.

Extensor pollicis longus

Origin: Ulna and interosseous membrane.
Insertion: Base of terminal phalanx of thumb.
Nerve supply: Posterior interosseous nerve.
Action: Extends phalanges and metacarpal of thumb.

Abductor pollicis brevis

Origin: From tubercle of scaphoid, ridge of trapezium, and flexor retinaculum.
Insertion: Outer side of base of proximal phalanx of thumb.
Nerve supply: Median nerve.
Action: Abducts the thumb.

Flexor pollicis brevis

Origin: Ridge of trapezium and flexor retinaculum.
Insertion: Outer side of base of proximal phalanx of thumb.
Nerve supply: Median nerve.
Action: Flexes proximal phalanx of thumb.

Opponens pollicis

Origin: Ridge of trapezium and flexor retinaculum.
Insertion: Radial side of metacarpal of thumb along whole length.
Nerve supply: Median nerve.
Action: Opposes thumb, i.e. brings the thumb over to the little finger.

Adductor pollicis

Origin: Transverse head: distal part of palmar surface of metacarpal of middle finger (third metacarpal). Oblique head: capitate, trapezoid, trapezium and metacarpals of index and middle fingers (second and third metacarpals).
Insertion: Inner side of proximal phalanx of thumb.
Nerve supply: Ulnar nerve (deep branch).
Action: Adducts the metacarpal of the thumb.

Abductor digiti minimi

Origin: Pisiform and flexor retinaculum.
Insertion: Medial side of base of proximal phalanx of little finger.
Nerve supply: Ulnar nerve.
Action: Abducts the little finger.

Flexor digiti minimi

Origin: Hook of the hamate and flexor retinaculum.
Insertion: Inserted with abductor digiti minimi into medial side of base of proximal phalanx of little finger.
Nerve supply: Ulnar nerve.
Action: Flexes and abducts the little finger.

Opponens digiti minimi

Origin: Hook of hamate and flexor retinaculum.
Insertion: Ulnar side of palmar aspect of metacarpal of little finger.
Nerve supply: Ulnar nerve.
Action: Opposes little finger with thumb.

Palmaris brevis

Origin: Palmar aponeurosis and flexor retinaculum.
Insertion: Skin on medial border of the hand.
Nerve supply: Ulnar nerve (superficial branch).
Action: Deepens the hollow in the palm of the hand.

The interossei and lumbricals of the hand

Four palmar interossei

Origin: Metacarpals of thumb, index, ring and little fingers.
Insertion: Side of base of proximal phalanx and extensor expansion. Thumb and index finger tendons run to ulnar side. Ring and little finger tendons run to radial side.
Nerve supply: Ulnar nerve (deep branch).
Action: Adduct the fingers and thumb. In addition they flex the metacarpophalangeal joints and extend the interphalangeal joints.

Four dorsal interossei

Origin: Two heads from adjacent metacarpals, e.g. thumb–index metacarpals.

Insertion: Side of base of proximal phalanx and extensor expansion. Index and one middle finger tendon run to radial side. Other middle finger tendon and ring finger tendon run to ulnar side.

Nerve supply: Ulnar nerve (deep branch)

Action: Abduct the index, middle and ring fingers at MCP joints. Also able to flex a straight finger.

Four lumbricals

Origin: From radial side of index tendon; from radial side of middle finger tendon; from adjacent sides of middle and ring finger; and from ring and little finger tendons.

Insertion: Radial side of extensor expansion of each finger.

Nerve supply: Median nerve: lateral two lumbricals. Ulnar nerve: medial two lumbricals.

Action: Flexes the metacarpophalangeal joints and extends the interphalangeal joints.

Multiple Choice Questions on the Upper Limb

1. Muscles taking part in the formation of the posterior wall of the axilla include:
(A) coracobrachialis
(B) short head of biceps
(C) latissimus dorsi
(D) teres major
(E) supraspinatus

A____ B____ C____ D____ E____

2. With respect to the muscles around the shoulder joint:
(A) infraspinatus produces medial rotation
(B) subscapularis is supplied by branches of the posterior cord of the brachial plexus
(C) supraspinatus is one of the tendinous cuff (rotator cuff) muscles
(D) deltoid is supplied by the axillary nerve
(E) latissimus dorsi is an adductor at the shoulder joint

A____ B____ C____ D____ E____

3. The axillary nerve contains fibres that carry:
(A) motor impulses to supraspinatus
(B) sensory impulses from skin on the lateral side of the upper arm
(C) motor impulses to the long head of triceps brachii
(D) sensory impulses from skin on the medial side of the upper arm
(E) motor impulses to subscapularis

A____ B____ C____ D____ E____

4. The serratus anterior muscle:
(A) is supplied by a branch of the medial cord of the brachial plexus
(B) lies in the medial wall of the axilla
(C) if paralysed: the scapula 'wings' when the limb pushes against resistance
(D) rotates the scapula on the chest wall
(E) attaches to the lateral border of the scapula

A____ B____ C____ D____ E____

5. The lateral cord of the brachial plexus:
(A) is found between the axillary artery and axillary vein
(B) gives a musculocutaneous branch
(C) gives a branch of supply to subscapularis
(D) has the ulnar nerve as a terminal branch
(E) supplies a branch to triceps

A____ B____ C____ D____ E____

6. Supraspinatus muscle:
(A) is separated from the shoulder joint by the subacromial bursa
(B) receives motor fibres from the dorsal scapular nerve
(C) contracts during abduction of the arm at the shoulder joint
(D) forms the superior boundary of the quadrangular space
(E) attaches to the greater tubercle of the humerus

A____ B____ C____ D____ E____

7. The deltoid muscle:
(A) is active during flexion of the shoulder joint
(B) is active during extension of the shoulder joint
(C) is a lateral rotator of the shoulder joint
(D) is supplied by a branch of the medial cord of the brachial plexus
(E) is attached to the greater tubercle of the humerus

A____ B____ C____ D____ E____

8. The synovial membrane of the shoulder joint:
(A) surrounds the long head of biceps brachii
(B) is continuous with the synovial membrane of the subacromial bursa
(C) surrounds the short head of biceps brachii
(D) lines the transverse humeral ligament
(E) surrounds the long head of triceps brachii

A____ B____ C____ D____ E____

9. During a radical mastectomy (surgical removal of the breast):
(A) the lateral group of axillary nodes will be found along the lower border of pectoralis minor
(B) the apical group of axillary nodes will be found at the medial side of the coracoid process
(C) lymph nodes will be found in association with the subscapular vessels
(D) the nerve to serratus anterior will be found in the posterior wall of the axilla
(E) damage to the nerve to latissimus dorsi will result in a winged scapula'

A____ B____ C____ D____ E____

10. The radial nerve:
(A) is a continuation of the posterior cord of the brachial plexus
(B) leaves the axilla through the quadrilateral space
(C) is accompanied by the posterior circumflex humeral artery
(D) supplies the triceps
(E) supplies the subscapularis

A____ B____ C____ D____ E____

11. The brachial plexus:
(A) is formed posterior to the scalenus medius muscle
(B) has four trunks
(C) gives radial and axillary nerves from its posterior cord
(D) is enclosed in a fascial sheath derived from the prevertebral fascia
(E) gives the long thoracic nerve from its medial cord

A____ B____ C____ D____ E____

12. The axillary nerve may be injured in a dislocation of the shoulder. Such an injury may be diagnosed by demonstrating impaired skin sensation over the:
(A) acromion
(B) upper half of the deltoid muscle
(C) lower half of the deltoid muscle
(D) spine of the scapula
(E) medial wall of the axilla

A____ B____ C____ D____ E____

13. Brachialis:
(A) lies deep to the biceps
(B) has the ulnar nerve between itself and biceps
(C) is supplied with motor fibres by the median nerve
(D) inserts into the coronoid process of the ulna
(E) forms the lateral border of the cubital fossa

A____ B ____ C ____ D ____ E ____

14. The radial artery:
(A) is formed in the cubital fossa
(B) may be located deep to brachioradialis in the forearm
(C) makes a contribution to the superficial palmar arch
(D) passes into the palm ultimately
(E) is located between the tendons of palmaris longus and flexor carpi radialis at the wrist

A____ B ____ C ____ D ____ E ____

15. The cubital fossa:
(A) is bounded partly by pronator teres
(B) has the supinator and brachialis in its floor
(C) has a roof which is reinforced by the bicipital aponeurosis
(D) contains the brachial artery on the medial side of the biceps tendon
(E) contains the ulnar nerve

A____ B ____ C ____ D ____ E ____

16. The anterior interosseous nerve:
(A) is a branch of the radial nerve
(B) supplies pronator teres
(C) supplies supinator
(D) supplies flexor pollicis longus
(E) supplies the lateral part of flexor digitorum profundus

A____ B ____ C ____ D ____ E ____

17. The ulnar nerve:
(A) is related to the back of the medial epicondyle at the elbow
(B) lies deep to flexor digitorum superficialis in the forearm
(C) supplies some fibres to flexor digitorum profundus
(D) supplies flexor pollicis longus
(E) supplies the pronator teres muscle

A____ B ____ C ____ D ____ E ____ .

18. With respect to the flexor aspect of the forearm:
(A) the palmaris longus passes deep to the flexor retinaculum
(B) the ulnar nerve runs along the medial edge of flexor digitorum superficialis
(C) brachioradialis is a flexor of the wrist
(D) pronator teres is supplied by the median nerve
(E) the tendon of flexor carpi radialis grooves the trapezium

A____ B ____ C ____ D ____ E ____

19. Supination of the forearm:
(A) turns the palm of the hand to face forwards in the anatomical position
(B) is produced by supinator when the elbow is held in full extension
(C) is impossible if the radial nerve is completely divided in the radial groove
(D) is a result of movements at two synovial joints
(E) can be produced by a muscle that arises from the scapula

A____ B ____ C ____ D ____ E ____

20. The tendon of extensor pollicis longus:
(A) passes deep to the extensor retinaculum
(B) possesses a synovial sheath
(C) forms one boundary of the anatomical snuffbox
(D) passes around the dorsal tubercle of the radius (Lister's tubercle)
(E) inserts into the base of the first (thumb) metacarpal

A____ B ____ C ____ D ____ E ____

21. Extensor carpi ulnaris:
(A) is supplied by the ulnar nerve
(B) runs deep to the extensor retinaculum
(C) contains a sesamoid bone
(D) will abduct the wrist joint in conjunction with flexor carpi ulnaris
(E) is attached to the lateral epicondyle of the humerus

A____ B ____ C ____ D ____ E ____

22. The scaphoid articulates with:
(A) the triquetrum
(B) the capitate
(C) the pisiform
(D) the lunate
(E) the trapezium

A____ B ____ C ____ D ____ E ____

23. The tendons of flexor digitorum superficialis:
(A) pass through the carpal tunnel
(B) have the median nerve on their lateral side within the carpal tunnel
(C) have the ulnar nerve on their medial side within the carpal tunnel
(D) are surrounded by synovial sheaths as they lie in the fibrous flexor sheaths of the fingers
(E) insert into the terminal phalanges of the fingers

A____ B ____ C ____ D ____ E ____

24. Concerning the anatomical snuff box:
(A) one boundary is the tendon of extensor pollicis longus
(B) the basilic vein is found in the overlying subcutaneous tissues
(C) the scaphoid can be palpated in its depths
(D) terminal branches of the radial nerve are found in the overlying subcutaneous tissues
(E) the radial artery may be palpated in the snuff box

A____ B ____ C ____ D ____ E ____

25. A laceration in the cubital fossa which completely severs the median nerve results in:
(A) claw hand
(B) paralysis of the muscles of the hypothenar eminence
(C) loss of sensation over the pulp of the thumb and index finger
(D) some loss of sensation in the palmar skin
(E) inability to flex the terminal interphalangeal joint of the index finger

A____ B ____ C ____ D ____ E ____

26. The ulnar nerve contains fibres that conduct:

(A) motor impulses to abductor pollicis brevis
(B) motor impulses to adduct the thumb
(C) motor impulses to flexor carpi ulnaris
(D) sensory impulses from the nail bed of the little finger
(E) motor impulses to abductor digiti minimi

A___ B ___ C ___ D ___ E ___

27. The median nerve contains fibres that conduct:

(A) motor impulses to opponens pollicis
(B) sensory impulses from the nail bed of the index finger
(C) motor impulses to flexor carpi radialis
(D) sensory impulses from the nail bed of the little finger
(E) motor impulses to opponens digiti minimi

A___ B ___ C ___ D ___ E ___

28. If the radial nerve is injured in the radial groove:

(A) the patient has wrist drop
(B) skin sensation is altered over the hypothenar eminence
(C) the medial two lumbrical muscles are paralysed
(D) the adductor pollicis is paralysed
(E) active extension at the metacarpophalangeal joints is impossible

A___ B ___ C ___ D ___ E ___

29. If the ulnar nerve is injured at the medial epicondyle of the humerus:

(A) there is muscle wasting and flattening of the thenar eminence of the thumb
(B) skin sensation is altered over the terminal phalanx of the index finger
(C) the muscles in the web between thumb and index finger are paralysed
(D) skin sensation is altered over the terminal phalanx of the little finger
(E) there is muscle wasting and flattening of the hypothenar eminence

A___ B ___ C ___ D ___ E ___

30. With respect to vessels in the upper limb:

(A) the basilic vein forms over the distal end of the radius
(B) the median cubital vein runs obliquely between the cephalic and basilic veins at the cubital fossa
(C) the radial and ulnar arteries each contribute to both the superficial and deep palmar arches in the hand
(D) the profunda brachii artery accompanies the radial nerve on the posterior aspect of the humerus
(E) the princeps pollicis is a branch of the superficial palmar arch

A___ B ___ C ___ D ___ E ___

Answers to Multiple Choice Questions

1.	AF BF CT DT EF	11.	AF BF CT DT EF	21.	AF BT CF DF ET
2.	AF BT CT DT ET	12.	AF BF CT DF EF	22.	AF BT CF DT ET
3.	AF BT CF DF EF	13.	AT BF CF DT EF	23.	AT BT CF DT EF
4.	AF BT CT DT EF	14.	AT BT CT DT EF	24.	AT BF CT DT ET
5.	AF BT CF DF EF	15.	AT BT CT DT EF	25.	AF BF CT DT ET
6.	AF BF CT DF ET	16.	AF BF CF DT ET	26.	AF BT CT DT ET
7.	AT BT CF DF EF	17.	AT BF CT DF EF	27.	AT BT CT DF EF
8.	AT BF CF DT EF	18.	AF BT CF DT ET	28.	AT BF CF DF ET
9.	AF BT CT DF EF	19.	AT BT CF DT ET	29.	AF BF CT DT ET
10.	AT BF CF DT EF	20.	AT BT CT DT EF	30.	AF BT CT DT EF

THE LOWER LIMB

The Front and Sides of the Thigh

The pelvic girdle both transmits the weight of the trunk to the lower limbs and provides a bony framework for the attachment of muscles that act on the proximal part of the lower limb. To study the thigh we need to look briefly at the bones that make up the pelvic girdle and then at the femur (Fig. 8.1).

Each hip or **innominate bone** develops from three separate bones called the **ilium**, the **pubis** and the **ischium** (Fig. 8.2). All three bones take part in the formation of a bony socket which forms part of the hip joint. This socket is called the **acetabulum**. In children each of these three bones can be seen on a radiograph, separated by cartilage. They join together within the acetabulum in a 'Y'-shaped configuration. Fusion of the three bones in this region occurs around puberty and the **triradiate cartilage** disappears just like an epiphyseal cartilage. This late fusion allows growth and adjustment of the acetabulum to continue in parallel with growth of the head of the femur.

In adults the acetabulum is a deep hemispherical bony socket. It takes part in the formation of the **hip joint** with the head of the femur. The parts of the **ilium** that are important to the study of the lower limb are the **iliac crest**, the **anterior superior** and **inferior iliac spines**. The iliac crest forms the rim of the ilium. It ends anteriorly as a bony prominence called the anterior superior iliac spine. Just below this is the anterior inferior iliac spine. These points are clearly seen when the bony pelvis is viewed from in front (Fig. 8.1). The iliac crest and anterior superior iliac spine are both easily palpable in the living subject.

Most of the pubic bone may also be seen in this view. The **superior** and **inferior pubic rami** meet at the body of the pubis. Stretching from the anterior superior iliac spine to the pubic tubercle on the body is the **inguinal ligament**. Review this structure: we will need to study the attachment of its medial end in more detail later.

The ischium can also be seen from this front view of the pelvis. The **ischial tuberosity** is clearly visible. The pubis and ischium surround an oval opening called the **obturator foramen**. More of the ischium is visible on a posterior view of the pelvis (Fig. 8.3).

The **ischial spine** is a pointed bony prominence. Above and below this point the bone is notched. Above it is the **greater sciatic notch** and below the smaller **lesser sciatic notch**. These notches are turned into foramina by two ligaments. The **sacrospinous ligament** extends from the ischial spine to the sacrum, and the **sacrotuberous ligament** from the ischial tuberosity to the sacrum and coccyx. The details of these two ligaments will also be studied later. Posteriorly, the **iliac crest** ends in the **posterior superior** and **posterior inferior iliac spines**. The posterior aspect of the **sacrum** and **coccyx** are visible from behind. The sacrum is wedged between the two pelvic bones, so forming the two **sacroiliac joints**.

Turn your attention now to the other bone that forms the hip joint, the femur. Its upper end presents a ball-shaped **head** and a narrow oblique **neck**. The head of the femur articulates with the acetabulum to form the 'ball and socket' hip joint. The head develops from a secondary ossification centre which appears during the first year of postnatal life. The growth and development of the head continues, and matches that of the acetabulum. Fusion of the head with the shaft occurs at about 16–18 years of age.

The angles made between the neck and shaft of the

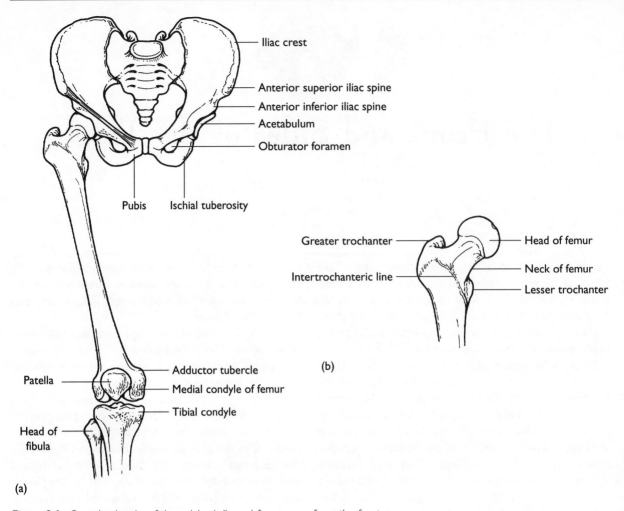

Figure 8.1   Bony landmarks of the pelvic girdle and femur seen from the front.

femur are important clinically (Fig. 8.4). The angle between the neck and the shaft of the femur is called the **angle of inclination**. It is normally somewhere between 116° and 140°. Many conditions, both congenital and acquired, may affect the angle of inclination. If the angle is diminished so that it is less than 116° the condition is known as **coxa vara**, whereas if the angle is increased to over 140° **coxa valga** is said to be present.

There is yet another angle to consider. This is the **angle of femoral torsion**. To understand this angle the femur should be viewed 'head on' from below (Fig. 8.5). The lower end of the femur is enlarged into two great **femoral condyles**. If a line is drawn through these condyles and the shaft eyed 'end on', it will be seen that the femoral neck does not project from the femur along this line but rather projects *anteromedi-*

ally. This angle of the femoral neck relative to the femoral condyles is the angle of femoral torsion. It is about 20° in the average femur. If this angle is altered then **torsion** of the femur is said to exist.

The upper end of the femoral shaft presents two large masses of bone called the **greater** and **lesser trochanters**. Viewed from the front, these two bony prominences are united by a line on the bone called the **intertrochanteric line** (Fig. 8.1). Behind, they are joined by a more marked **intertrochanteric crest** of bone. A fossa exists in the back of the greater trochanter, at the root of this crest, and is called the **trochanteric fossa** (Fig. 8.3). The front of the **shaft** of the femur presents no important landmarks, but on the back of the shaft there is a long rough crest of bone called the **linea aspera**. Above, the linea aspera divides and runs into the **spiral line** more medially and the

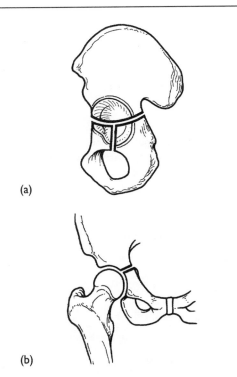

(a)

(b)

Figure 8.2 (a) The triradiate cartilage divides the innominate bone into ilium, pubis and ischium. (b) The ilium transmits the weight of the trunk to the head of the femur.

gluteal tuberosity laterally (Fig. 8.3). Below, it divides into two **supracondylar lines**.

We saw in the upper limb that all nerves and vessels entered the arm through the axilla and then ran into either flexor or extensor compartments. In the case of the lower limb, nerves and vessels enter the thigh in one of three ways.

One entrance is for the **femoral nerve** and vessels that travel to the front of the thigh. Most of the muscles on the front of the thigh extend the knee joint. The nerves and vessels approach this region through the elongated interval between the inguinal ligament and the bone of the pelvis below it (Fig. 8.6). The second port of entry is for the nerve and vessels that travel to the medial aspect of the thigh. The group of muscles in this region are the adductor muscles of the hip joint (Fig. 8.7). The **obturator nerve** and vessels enter and leave this part of the thigh through the **obturator foramen**. The third entrance is best seen on a posterior view of the pelvis. It is for the nerve that travels to the posterior aspect of the leg. This is the **sciatic nerve**, which travels to the back of the thigh through the **greater sciatic for-**

amen. In the back of the thigh the sciatic nerve supplies the flexor muscles of the knee (Fig. 8.8).

The thigh can be usefully subdivided for study into the following regions. The front and sides of the thigh are best studied first and then the **gluteal region** (Fig. 8.9). Next it makes sense to study the hip joint so that its movements and important relationships may be learned quickly. Finally, attention can be turned to the back of the thigh and to the structures behind the knee in the so-called **popliteal region**.

Look at the muscles on the medial side of the thigh and then at the great mass of musculature on the front of the thigh. The muscles along the medial side of the femur are powerful **adductors** of the hip joint. Most of them are supplied by the **obturator nerve**. The muscles also have a weak rotational pull on the femur. This adductor mass forms a flat, muscular septum on the medial side of the thigh (Fig. 8.10). It is a fairly complete muscular septum except for a 'hole' in its lower reaches.

On the lateral side of the femur there is a fibrous septum. This extends from the linea aspera at the back of the femur. It stretches outwards between the muscles to the deep fascia of the thigh. This sheet of fascia is called the **lateral intermuscular septum**. The **adductor muscle sheet**, the **shaft of the femur** and the **lateral intermuscular septum** together form a **musculo-osseofascial partition** stretching across the thigh. In front of the partition lies the **extensor mass** for the knee and behind it the **flexor mass** of musculature.

Now we can look at the **adductor muscles** in a little more detail. They arise from the ischium and pubis, and stretch to the back of the femur. They are arranged in three strata and can adduct and/or medially rotate the femur at the hip joint. The deepest stratum is the bulkiest and most complete, being made up largely from a vast muscle called the **adductor magnus** (Figs 8.10 and 8.11). This muscle arises from the ischial tuberosity and part of the inferior pubic ramus. It is the thickest portion of the muscle and is inserted low down on the femoral shaft into an elevation called the **adductor tubercle**. The rest of the muscle is inserted into the supracondylar ridge and linea aspera. In the lower part of the muscle there is an elongated gap. The femoral vessels pass through this passageway as they travel between the front of the thigh and back of the knee. The adductor magnus muscle adducts the femur at the hip joint. It is supplied by the **obturator nerve**. The lower part of the muscle can also weakly extend the thigh as well as

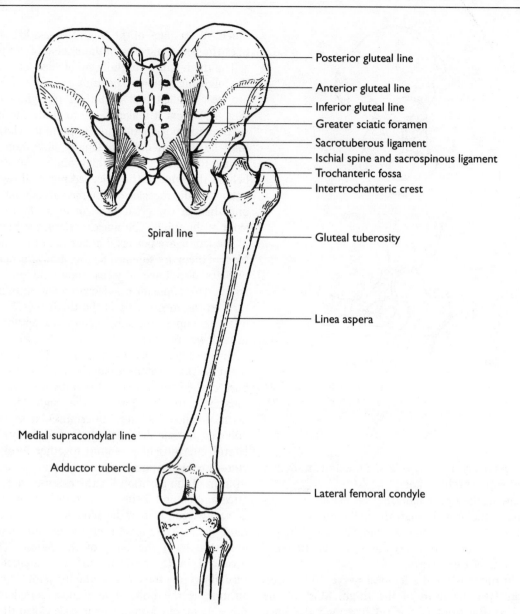

Posterior gluteal line

Anterior gluteal line

Inferior gluteal line

Greater sciatic foramen

Sacrotuberous ligament

Ischial spine and sacrospinous ligament

Trochanteric fossa

Intertrochanteric crest

Spiral line

Gluteal tuberosity

Linea aspera

Medial supracondylar line

Adductor tubercle

Lateral femoral condyle

Figure 8.3 Bony landmarks of the pelvic girdle and femur seen from behind.

adducting it. In fact the fibres that do this are supplied from behind by the sciatic nerve.

A long slender muscle skirts the side of the adductor group. It is the **gracilis**. It extends from the pubis, beyond the knee joint, to the tibia. It therefore spans two joints, the hip joint and the knee (Fig. 8.10). The muscle is an adductor of the thigh but also can flex the knee joint. It is suppled by the obturator nerve.

The **obturator externus** muscle arises from the external surface of the obturator membrane and the surrounding bone around the lower part of the obtu-

rator foramen. It passes below the neck of the femur and capsule of the hip joint, curves up over the back of the joint, and inserts into the floor of the **trochanteric fossa**. Since it is attached so close to the joint it has no adducting ability, but its mechanical pull makes it an efficient lateral rotator. It is supplied by the obturator nerve.

The middle stratum of muscle on the medial aspect of the thigh is small and represented by one muscle only, the **adductor brevis** (Fig. 8.11). This muscle arises from the pubic arch below the symphysis and

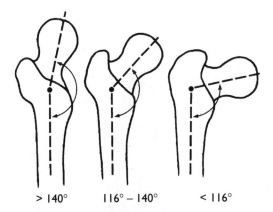

Figure 8.4 The angle of inclination between the neck and shaft of the femur is usually between 116° and 140°. In coxa vara it is diminished and in coxa valga it is in excess of 140°.

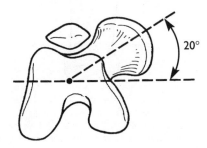

Figure 8.5 The angle of femoral torsion between the femoral condyles and the femoral neck is about 20°.

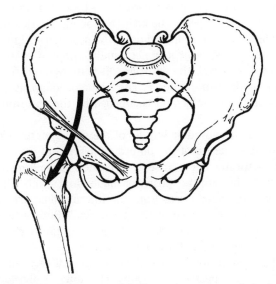

Figure 8.6 The course of the femoral nerve beneath the inguinal ligament into the front of the thigh.

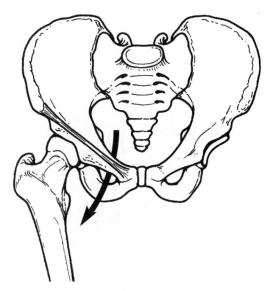

Figure 8.7 The course of the obturator nerve through the obturator foramen of the pelvis into the medial aspect of the thigh.

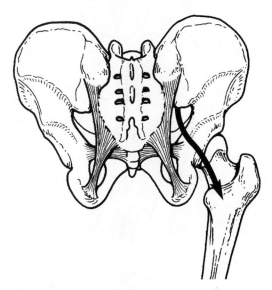

Figure 8.8 The course of the sciatic nerve through the greater sciatic foramen and into the back of the thigh.

fans out to its insertion at the linea aspera on the back of the femur. Adductor brevis is an adductor of the femur and is supplied by the obturator nerve.

The superficial layer of muscles is made up of two muscles, the **pectineus** and the **adductor longus**. These are each triangular in shape, the **pectineus** arising from the pubis by its **base** and the **adductor longus** from the body of the pubis by its **apex**. They are both flat muscles and pass side by side to the back of the

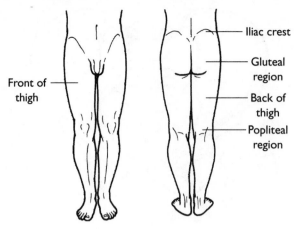

Figure 8.9   The front, sides and back of the thigh.

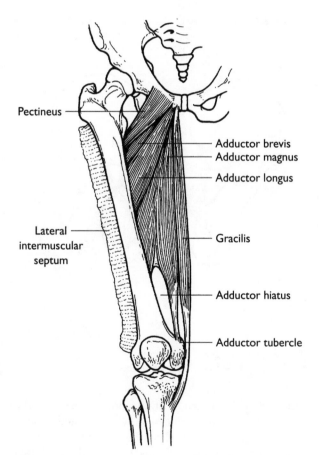

Figure 8.10   The adductor musculature on the medial side of the thigh.

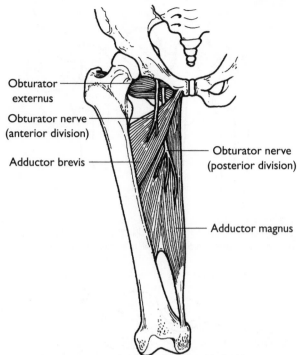

Figure 8.11   The anterior division of the obturator nerve passes over the top of obturator externus. The posterior division pierces the middle of obturator externus. Adductor longus, in fact, overlies adductor brevis and adductor magnus superiorly and is not shown in this diagram.

femur (Fig. 8.10). The pectineus is inserted by a short tendon on to the bone between the lesser trochanter and the linea aspera. The adductor longus inserts into the linea aspera itself. Although the pectineus is functionally an *adductor* it is *not* usually supplied by the 'adductor nerve', the obturator. It is more often supplied by the femoral nerve. The adductor longus is an important adductor and is supplied by the obturator nerve.

The neurovascular bundle of the adductor muscle mass is made up of the obturator nerve and vessels. The obturator nerve arises as a branch of the **lumbar plexus** high in the posterior abdominal wall. The **obturator artery** arises from the internal iliac artery on the inner surface of the pelvic wall. Both artery and nerve enter the medial side of the thigh by passing through the **obturator foramen**.

The obturator nerve divides immediately into anterior and posterior divisions. The anterior division passes over the upper border of the obturator externus to gain the interval between the superficial and middle layers of adductor muscles. It supplies the longus, brevis, pectineus and gracilis. The posterior division pierces the obturator externus and descends between the intermediate and deep layers of the adductor mass. It supplies the obturator externus and the magnus. The obturator artery also divides into anterior and posterior divisions but these simply form an arterial mesh on the obturator membrane. More important is an arterial branch from the posterior division. This passes through the acetabular notch to supply blood to the head of the femur. We will discuss it further during our the study of the hip joint.

Look now at the extensor mass of musculature which lies in front of the musculo-osseofascial partition (Fig. 8.12) in the thigh. Be very clear in your mind that these muscles are *mostly* extensors of the *knee joint, not* the hip joint. Many students become confused with the movements of the two joints. Notice that, since the adductor sheet and the lateral intermuscular septum both attach to the back of the femur, there is room for this great extensor mass to clothe both the front and sides of the femoral shaft. The great extensor of the knee is a compound muscle called the **quadriceps femoris**. The quadriceps, as its name implies, is composed of four parts, the **vastus medialis**, **vastus intermedius** and **vastus lateralis** and a more superficial part called the **rectus femoris**. In the distal part of the thigh all four bellies become tendinous and unite to form a strong **common tendon of the quadriceps** (Fig. 8.12). The tendon is inserted into the patella and continues to be anchored into the tibial tuberosity by means of the **ligamentum patellae**. The patella is in fact a sesamoid bone and if necessary it may be removed without interfering with extension of the knee joint. Such a procedure is sometimes required following a very badly fractured patella.

Several **bursae** may be found around the patella. They facilitate movement of the skin over the patella and tibial tuberosity, and of the common tendon on the underlying bone (Fig. 8.13). The **prepatellar bursa** is found just deep to the skin in front of the lower part of the patella. A chronic enlargement of this bursa from the oft-repeated trauma of kneeling gives rise to the condition known as 'housemaid's knee'. A subcutaneous **infrapatellar bursa** lies deep to the skin over the upper part of the tibia. Two deep bursae are also associated with the extensor apparatus. A **deep infrapatellar bursa** lies between the ligamentum patellae and the tibia, and so prevents friction here during movement of the knee. The **suprapatellar bursa** is an extension of the synovial membrane of the knee joint.

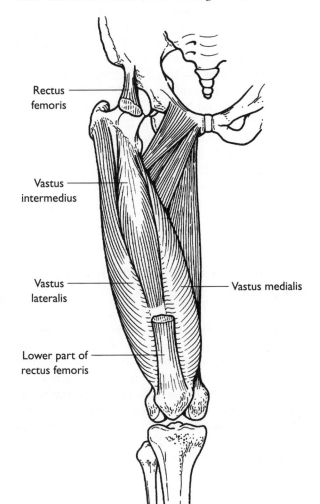

Rectus femoris

Vastus intermedius

Vastus lateralis

Vastus medialis

Lower part of rectus femoris

Figure 8.12 The quadriceps form the extensor muscles of the knee joint in front of the musculo-osseofascial partition of the thigh.

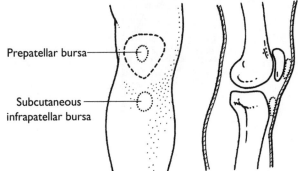

Prepatellar bursa

Subcutaneous infrapatellar bursa

Figure 8.13 The prepatellar and infrapatellar bursae facilitate movement of the skin over the patella, patellar ligament and tibial tuberosity.

It insinuates itself up between the common tendon and the front of the femur.

Of the four parts of the quadriceps, the **vastus intermedius** arises from a large area on the front and sides of the femoral shaft. The **medialis** and **lateralis** have linear origins on either side towards the back of the shaft of the femur, mainly from the linea aspera. The superficial belly of the muscle, the **rectus femoris**, lies on the surface of the other bellies. It arises from the **pelvis** and not from the femur like the other parts of the muscle. Rectus femoris arises from the anterior inferior iliac spine and from the bone just above the acetabulum (Fig. 8.14).

The action of the quadriceps is to **extend** the knee joint. Since the rectus femoris also arises from the pelvis and spans the hip joint, this head may also act as a hip flexor. The nerve supply to quadriceps is the **femoral nerve**. Two other muscles appear in the proximal part of the thigh. These large muscle masses arise in the abdominopelvic cavity and converge as a common tendon on to the lesser trochanter of the femur. They are **flexors** of the hip joint, and are the **psoas major** and the **iliacus**. Both muscles are supplied by the femoral nerve. The muscles pass deep to the inguinal ligament to reach the lesser trochanter. The iliacus is fleshy in its entire course whereas the psoas fibres give rise to a strong tendon as it approaches the insertion. The iliacus muscle inserts both into the tendon of psoas and into the bone of the lesser trochanter. The combined iliopsoas muscle and its tendon pass over the front of the capsule of the hip joint. They are often separated from it by a bursa. This allows free movement of the tendon on the joint capsule. Both psoas and iliacus are flexors of the thigh at the hip joint but psoas is also a medial rotator of the thigh when it is in the flexed position.

We can complete our study of the muscles of the front of the thigh by looking at a long, narrow muscle called the **sartorius**. Sartorius arises from the anterior superior iliac spine and crosses obliquely in front of the thigh to extend below the knee joint. Here it is inserted into the medial side of the tibia. It is a flexor of both the hip and knee joints and also laterally rotates the thigh. This is the muscle we use when taking up a cross-legged sitting position on the floor. It was for this reason that it was called the 'sartorius' or the tailor's muscle. It is supplied by the femoral nerve (Fig. 8.15).

The femoral triangle and femoral canal

Look carefully at Figure 8.15, noting the pattern formed by the muscles on the front of the thigh. A 'triangle' can be identified whose base is the **inguinal ligament**. The two sides of the triangle are formed by the **sartorius** laterally and the medial border of the **adductor longus**, **pectineus** and the insertions of the **psoas** and **iliacus**. Superficially the triangle is covered with **deep fascia** fat and skin. This triangle is called the **femoral triangle**.

The apex of the femoral triangle leads to an intermuscular cleft which lies between the **vastus medialis** and the **adductor magnus**. It is covered superficially by the **sartorius**. At the distal end of the intermuscular cleft is the elongated opening we noted above in the adductor magnus. The intermuscular cleft is

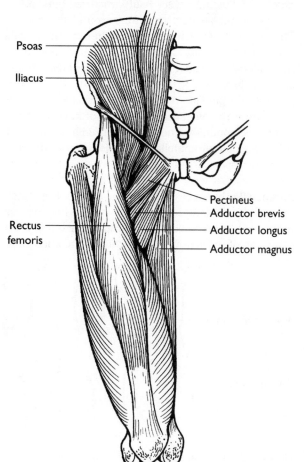

Psoas
Iliacus
Rectus femoris
Pectineus
Adductor brevis
Adductor longus
Adductor magnus

Figure 8.14   Psoas, iliacus and rectus femoris.

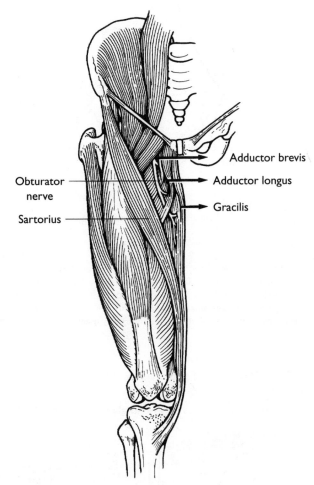

The femoral nerve is a branch of the **lumbar plexus**. It also enters the limb by passing behind the inguinal ligament. Lymphatics from the limb follow the femoral artery into the abdominopelvic cavity and then travel eventually along the para-aortic channels. It is best to follow each of these neurovascular structures as they pass through three regions of the thigh. First we need to note how they enter or leave the limb behind the inguinal ligament. Next we must follow their course and distribution in the femoral triangle, and finally we need to understand their passage through the adductor canal (Fig. 8.16, arrow).

To understand the passage of these neurovascular structures behind the inguinal ligament we need to review the anatomy of the **inguinal ligament** itself. It is especially important now to remember the **lacunar ligament**. This little triangular ligament fills in the medial end of the oval space between the inguinal ligament and the **pecten pubis**. The lateral edge of the lacunar ligament presents a sharp edge (Fig. 8.17).

The femoral nerve is formed in the substance of the psoas muscle as part of the lumbar plexus. It remains in close contact with the iliopsoas muscle as it passes behind the inguinal ligament. The femoral artery and

Figure 8.15 The sartorius laterally, the medial border of adductor longus medially and the inguinal ligament above, form what is known as the femoral triangle on the anterior aspect of the thigh.

called the **adductor canal**. Roughly half way down the thigh the sartorius muscle overlies the adductor longus and forms the so-called **subsartorial canal** beneath it.

Having studied the muscles on the front of the thigh, we can look next at the vessels, nerves and lymphatics in this region. The arterial supply to the lower limb is derived from the **femoral artery**. This is a continuation of the external iliac artery and it enters the limb by passing behind the inguinal ligament. The venous blood from the lower limb collects eventually into an accompanying vein called the **femoral vein**. This becomes the external iliac vein as it enters the abdominopelvic cavity behind the inguinal ligament. The nerve of this compartment is the **femoral nerve**.

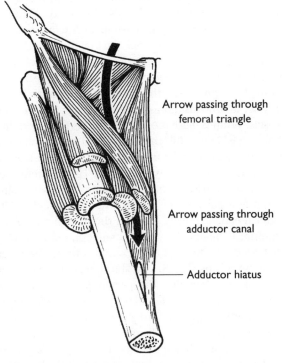

Figure 8.16 The course of the femoral nerve and vessels through the femoral triangle, adductor canal and adductor hiatus.

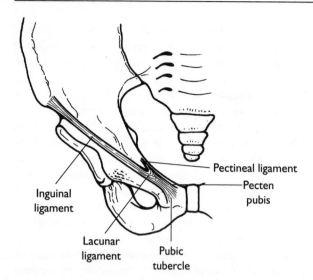

Figure 8.17 The inguinal ligament spans the gap between the anterior superior iliac spine and the pubic tubercle. The lacunar ligament forms the medial boundary of the femoral ring. The pectineal ligament runs on below this to attach to the pecten pubis.

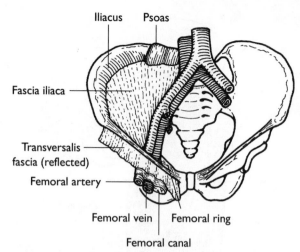

Figure 8.18 The femoral canal, femoral vein and femoral artery are surrounded in front by an extension of fascia transversalis (seen here reflected forwards from the inguinal ligament) and by an extension of fascia iliaca behind. This so-called femoral sheath extends for about one inch into the thigh.

vein on the other hand are enclosed in a condensation of fascia as they pass behind the inguinal ligament. This fascia is called the **femoral sheath**. It extends around the vessels for about one inch into the thigh and blends with the vessel walls. The femoral sheath is said to be formed by extensions of **fascia transversalis** which form the anterior part of the sheath and the **fascia iliaca** which form the posterior aspect. This is a rather idealistic view and, in fact, in the operating room the femoral sheath can really be demonstrated only as a condensation of areolar tissue around the vessels. What is *much* more important is to realize that the vessels do not 'fill' the medial end of the oval gap next to the lacunar ligament (Fig. 8.18). This is filled with a little fat and a lymph node. This collection of loose areolar tissue which lies along the medial side of the femoral vein for almost one inch is called the **femoral canal**. Directly beneath the medial end of the inguinal ligament the canal is surrounded by a ring of structures. This part of the canal is therefore called the **femoral ring** (Fig. 8.19). The ring is formed by the femoral vein laterally, the pecten pubis posteriorly, the sharp edge of the lacunar ligament medially and the inguinal ligament anteriorly. Trace the boundaries of this ring on the diagram. Be clear at this point that you realize that the femoral artery lies lateral to the femoral vein as they both pass beneath the inguinal ligament (Fig. 8.18). The femoral canal is

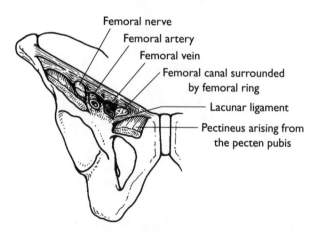

Figure 8.19 The femoral canal is surrounded by a ring of structures: the lacunar ligament medially, the pecten pubis posteriorly, the femoral vein laterally and the inguinal ligament anteriorly.

important since, under certain conditions, abdominal contents push through the femoral ring and easily squeeze along the fatty femoral canal. They then bulge out into the superficial tissues of the thigh and present as a swelling called a **femoral hernia** (see below).

Each of the neurovascular structures may now be traced into the femoral triangle. The femoral artery emerges from behind the inguinal ligament at the **femoral point**. This can be marked on the skin as a position midway between the symphysis pubis and the anterior superior iliac spine. The femoral artery is covered by the fascia of the femoral sheath and is the most lateral of the three structures surrounded by the sheath (artery, vein and femoral canal). The fascia of the sheath soon fuses and blends with the walls of the vessel. The femoral nerve is on the lateral side of the artery, but not included in the fascia of the sheath. The nerve, however, does not follow the artery for long since it quickly breaks up into many branches (Fig. 8.20).

The femoral artery and vein

The femoral artery passes through the femoral triangle towards its apex. However, while still in the triangle it gives off a very large branch called the **profunda femoris**. This vessel is often as large as the femoral artery itself and is the principal blood vessel supplying the thigh. Its function is to supply much of the musculature of the thigh. It arises in the proximal part of the triangle, curves behind the parent artery, and dips deeply between the two superficial adductor muscles, the pectineus and adductor longus. **Lateral** and **medial circumflex branches** arise from the profunda soon after it is formed. The lateral is larger and

passes to the deep surface of the rectus femoris. It sends ascending branches up to the hip region for the supply of muscles and the hip joint itself, and transverse branches into the vasti which also course around the back of the femur. Descending branches pass down to the musculature of the knee region. The medial circumflex artery sinks into the medial side of the thigh musculature over the upper border of the adductor magnus. It also gives ascending branches to the hip region and transverse branches to the muscles at the back of the thigh, some of which anastomose behind the femur with branches of the lateral circumflex artery. A typical plan of arterial supply from the profunda artery is shown in Figure 8.21; however, do not be surprised to find variations. **Perforating branches** of the profunda pierce and supply the adductor sheet, then travel around the back of the femur to supply the muscles of the posterior compartment. They end by supplying much of the great vastus lateralis mass.

Four small superficial branches of the femoral artery are found soon after it has passed into the femoral triangle. These fan out to surrounding superficial tissues. They are accompanied by veins and their only

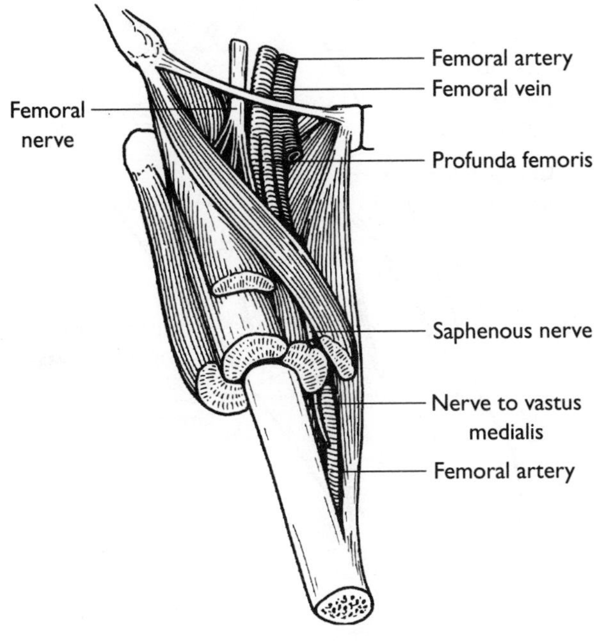

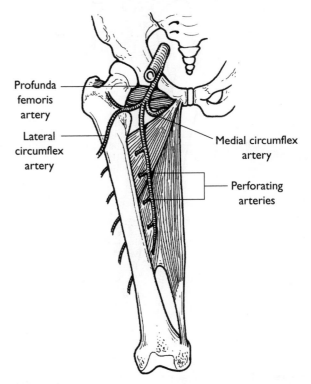

Figure 8.20 The femoral nerve and femoral vessels in the femoral triangle.

Figure 8.21 Typical branches of the profunda femoris artery in the thigh.

'claim to fame' is that the veins are important in the treatment of varicose veins (see below). The femoral vein lies on the medial side of the artery in the femoral sheath. It passes up alongside the femoral artery from the apex of the femoral triangle. As the two vessels travel through the femoral triangle they spiral in such a way that, towards the apex of the femoral triangle, the vein passes behind the artery (Fig. 8.22). The vein becomes the external iliac vein as soon as it passes behind the inguinal ligament. The tributaries of the vein do not exactly correspond to the branches of the artery. The **profunda vein** usually runs with the artery of the same name, but the **lateral** and **medial circumflex veins** often enter the femoral vein directly.

The femoral vein receives in its superficial part a large and important superficial vein called the **great saphenous vein**. This long vein originates on the medial side of the foot and ankle and drains blood from the medial side of the leg and thigh. It runs in

the subcutaneous fat of the leg and eventually reaches the front of the thigh just below the inguinal ligament. Here it lies directly over the femoral vein. However, to reach the femoral vein it has to pierce the thick, tough **deep fascia** of the thigh (Fig. 8.23). This deep fascia is given the name **fascia lata**. The great saphenous vein dips deeply to enter the femoral vein through an opening in the fascia lata called the **saphenous opening**. This opening contains only a little loose areolar tissue which is called the **cribriform fascia**.

Before entering the femoral vein, the great saphenous vein receives four tributaries. Their names are given in Figure 8.23, but they need not be memorized. They have the same names as accompanying branches of the femoral artery. They gain importance only during the treatment of varicose veins. The great saphenous vein contains many **valves** since it lies in the subcutaneous fat and therefore cannot rely on muscle action to aid the flow of blood through it. If these valves cease to function and the pressure rises in the vein, stagnation and pooling of blood occurs. The vein then becomes dilated and tortuous. The con-

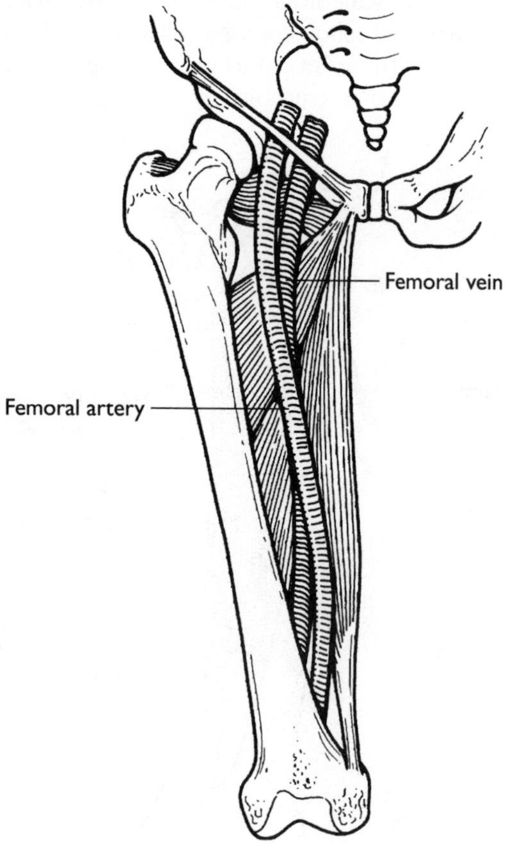

Figure 8.22 The femoral vein and artery spiral past one another so that the vein comes to lie behind the artery at the apex of the femoral triangle.

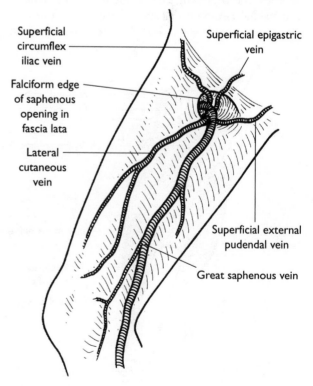

Figure 8.23 Venous tributaries of the great saphenous vein converging on the saphenous opening in the fascia lata.

dition is known as **varicose veins**. In the lower leg and ankle the vein communicates with deep veins, these communications being known simply as **perforators**.

The femoral nerve does not have a long course in the femoral triangle. It enters the triangle behind the inguinal ligament. Here it accompanies the iliopsoas muscle and tendon. It lies to the lateral side of the femoral artery outside the femoral sheath (Fig. 8.20). It soon ends in the proximal part of the triangle by dividing into a leash of terminal branches. It gives **cutaneous branches** to the skin on the front of the thigh and a long cutaneous nerve called the **saphenous nerve** which accompanies the femoral artery to the apex of the femoral triangle.

The muscular branches of the femoral nerve supply the pectineus, sartorius and all parts of the quadriceps femoris. The branch to the vastus medialis is long and accompanies the femoral artery to the apex of the femoral triangle. The nerve also supplies branches to both hip and knee joints. The femoral nerve is not the

only branch of the lumbar plexus to reach the front of the thigh. The **lateral cutaneous nerve of the thigh** is one branch that passes into the subcutaneous tissues of the thigh. It appears from behind the most lateral end of the inguinal ligament (Fig. 8.24). It is occasionally irritated by pressure from the ligament such that cutaneous pain is felt on the outer surface of the thigh. The **genitofemoral nerve** is another branch of the lumbar plexus. After giving off the genital branch it continues behind the inguinal ligament and emerges to supply a small area of skin below the ligament.

The **ilioinguinal nerve**, after escaping through the superficial inguinal ring, supplies the skin on the scrotum or labia majora. It also supplies skin on the adjacent part of the thigh. If this nerve is injured during operation to correct inguinal hernia, the patient often complains of loss of sensation in the area of skin supplied by the nerve.

The **lymph nodes** in the femoral triangle are important filter stations for lymph from the lower

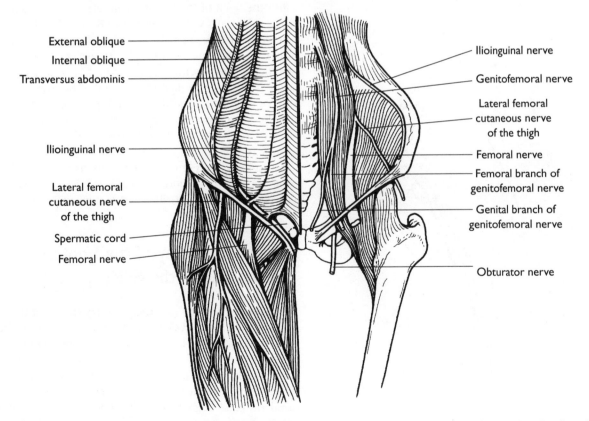

Figure 8.24 The relationship of the nerves of the lumbar plexus to the muscle layers of the anterior abdominal wall and medial aspect of the thigh in a male.

limb. They are arranged in superficial and deep groups. The **superficial inguinal lymph nodes** are arranged like a letter 'T' (Fig. 8.25). The vertically arranged nodes are found around the great saphenous vein. The horizontally arranged nodes lie in the subcutaneous fat below the inguinal ligament. These nodes receive lymph from the superficial layers of the limb, buttock and external genitalia as well as from the perineum and lower part of the anterior abdominal wall. Efferents from these nodes pass to the **deep inguinal lymph nodes**. These are found surrounding the femoral vein. One node of this group is quite consistently found in the fat of the femoral canal. Efferents from these deep inguinal nodes drain into the external iliac nodes through lymphatic channels which pass behind the inguinal ligament. It is normal to be able to palpate a few inguinal nodes even in a healthy individual.

In summary, we can say therefore that the **femoral triangle** is a region bounded by the inguinal ligament above and the sartorius and adductor longus below. These two muscles meet at the apex of the triangle.

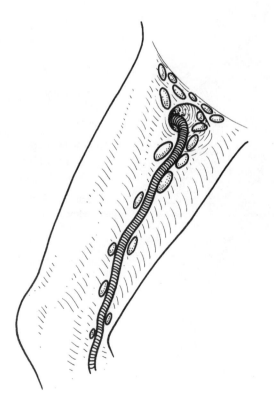

Figure 8.25 The superficial inguinal lymph nodes in the thigh are arranged in the form of a letter 'T'.

The triangle contains the **femoral vessels, profunda vessels** and their branches as well as the **femoral nerve** and its branches. Around the vein are the **deep inguinal lymph nodes**. Superficially, the triangle is covered by dense **fascia lata** in which there is a **saphenous opening**. In the subcutaneous tissues overlying the triangle are cutaneous nerves and the great saphenous vein. These are surrounded by superficial lymph nodes.

Now we can study the passage of these neurovascular structures through the **adductor canal**. The adductor canal lies between the vastus medialis and the adductor magnus (Fig. 8.16). At the distal end of the canal is the hiatus in the adductor magnus. The canal is roofed superficially by a layer of fascia and by the sartorius muscle. The femoral artery passes through the adductor canal and out of the apex of the femoral triangle into the hiatus. From here it passes to the posterior aspect of the knee through the hiatus, where it is renamed the **popliteal artery**. The popliteal vein also enters the adductor canal through the hiatus. It is renamed the **femoral vein** as it passes anteriorly into the apex of the femoral triangle. In this position it lies lateral to the artery (Fig. 8.22). The femoral nerve is largely spent by the time it approaches the apex of the femoral triangle. However, two of its branches travel with the artery and vein part of the way through the adductor canal. The **saphenous nerve** passes through the canal to emerge on the side of the knee where it joins the great saphenous vein. It is destined to supply sensation to the skin in the lower reaches of the leg. The **nerve to vastus medialis** is also to be seen entering the canal as it approaches the apex of the femoral triangle. While in the canal it sends branches into the vastus medialis muscle.

Applied anatomy of the front and medial side of the thigh

A **quadriceps reflex** (or **knee-jerk reflex**) is routinely elicited during physical examination. Tapping the patellar ligament briskly results in the immediate reflex extension of the leg at the knee joint. Muscle spindles in the quadriceps are first stretched, then afferent impulses from these spindles travel in the femoral nerve to segments L2, L3 and L4 of the spinal cord. From here, impulses are transmitted via a second sensory axon within the spinal cord to motor

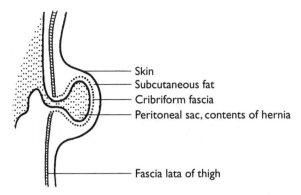

Figure 8.26 Cross-section through a femoral hernia that has protruded through the saphenous opening in the fascia lata of the thigh.

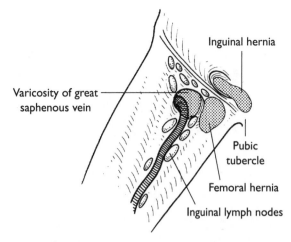

Figure 8.27 Some possible structures that can give rise to swellings in the medial part of the thigh.

or efferent fibres that travel back to the quadriceps muscle. Absence of a quadriceps reflex can result from any lesion that interrupts this reflex arc. A good example would be a herniated intervertebral disc that is protruding into the vertebral canal.

Fractures of the shaft of the femur are not uncommon. So too are fractures of the patella or ruptures of the rectus femoris muscle in young athletes, or of the tendon in older patients. One of the most important things to consider in this region is **femoral hernia**. Here, bowel or omentum, covered with parietal peritoneum, passes through the femoral ring into the femoral canal. At this point the hernia is small. The abdominal protrusion, in its peritoneal sac, can pass along the whole length of the femoral canal. It then finds itself deep to the saphenous opening in the fascia lata (Fig. 8.23). Here it is free to balloon

through this hole into the subcutaneous fat of the thigh. In so doing, it gains another 'sac' to cover itself, in the form of the cribriform fascia. Such a hernia now presents as a swelling in the groin (Fig. 8.26).

It is a good anatomical exercise to list some of the other possible structures that can present as a swelling in this region when they become abnormal (Fig. 8.27). Lymph nodes, for example, may enlarge and become painful. Varicosities of the great saphenous vein as it dips through the saphenous opening can occasionally cause a swelling in the groin. An abscess, formed in the lumbar vertebral region, will sometimes track down the psoas sheath and present as a swelling in the groin since the insertion of the muscle is in this region (Fig. 8.14).

chapter
9

The Gluteal Region and the Hip Joint

The great mass of muscle that makes up the buttock or gluteal region takes origin from the bony pelvis and lies both above and behind the hip joint. The skeletal framework of the region is made up of the posterior aspects of the **sacrum**, **pelvis** and upper or proximal end of the **femur** (Fig. 9.1).

Two important ligaments transform what are essentially bony notches into two foramina. The ligaments are the **sacrotuberous** and the **sacrospinous** ligaments. The sacrotuberous ligament extends from the ischial tuberosity to both posterior iliac spines and to the margins of the sacrum and coccyx. Partly hidden under cover of the sacrotuberous ligament is the sacrospinous ligament. This arises from the spine of

the ischium and stretches to the pelvic surface of the sacrum and coccyx. It is, in fact, nothing more than the superficial fibrous part of the **coccygeus muscle** which has virtually no function in humans. The upper foramen is called the **greater sciatic foramen**. Terminal branches of the **sacral plexus** stream out through this hole in company with blood vessels and a muscle called **piriformis**. The nerves that leave through this foramen are destined to supply the back of the leg and the buttock. The lower of the two foramina is called the **lesser sciatic foramen**. It is both a point of entry into the perineum and a path of exit for the **obturator internus** muscle which is destined for the hip joint. The nerve of the perineum and its

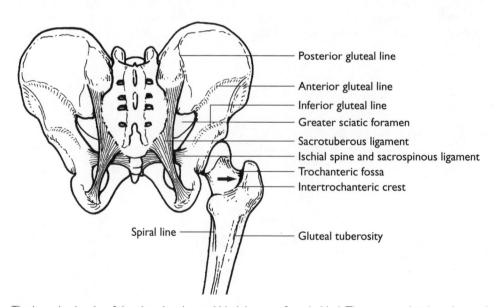

Figure 9.1 The bony landmarks of the gluteal region and hip joint seen from behind. The arrow points into the trochanteric fossa.

Labels (top to bottom, right side):
- Posterior gluteal line
- Anterior gluteal line
- Inferior gluteal line
- Greater sciatic foramen
- Sacrotuberous ligament
- Ischial spine and sacrospinous ligament
- Trochanteric fossa
- Intertrochanteric crest
- Gluteal tuberosity

Label (left side): Spiral line

accompanying blood vessels leave the abdominopelvic cavity through the greater sciatic foramen. They then curl around the ischial spine and sacrospinous complex, and enter the perineum.

Three roughened bony markings, the **posterior**, **anterior** and **inferior gluteal lines** divide up the outer surface of the ilium in this view (Fig. 9.1). These markings represent the origins of the great gluteal muscles on the bone. The posterior aspect of the hip joint is most clear in this view. Between the greater and lesser trochanters at the back of the femur is a raised **intertrochanteric crest**. The **trochanteric fossa** lies medial to the crest in the medial aspect of the greater trochanter. Just below the greater trochanter, there is a roughened **gluteal tuberosity** that runs down to the **linea aspera**. The muscles of the gluteal region can be divided into three functional groups. The first functional group of muscles clothe the posterior aspect of the hip joint. These are the **lateral rotators** of the femur at the hip joint. One of these muscles arises from inside the pelvis and therefore enters the region through the greater sciatic foramen. Another arises mainly from the side wall of the perineum and therefore enters the hip region through the lesser sciatic foramen. They are the **piriformis** and the **obturator internus** muscles respectively (Figs 9.2 and 9.3).

The **piriformis** arises from the pelvic surface of the middle three fused segments of the sacrum and passes directly out through the greater sciatic foramen. In the gluteal region it tapers rapidly, giving rise to a tendon, which inserts into the greater trochanter high

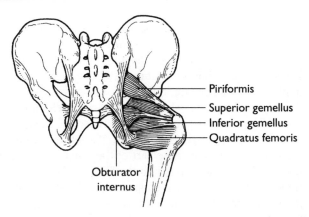

Figure 9.3 The lateral rotators of the hip joint seen from behind.

up. It is supplied by branches of the sacral plexus and is a **lateral rotator** of the hip. The **obturator internus** arises from the internal surface of the obturator membrane and bone surrounding the obturator foramen. Its tendon converges on to the lesser sciatic foramen where it hooks around the lesser sciatic notch. The notch acts as a pulley, the tendon turning at right angles around it. To reduce friction here, there is a bursa separating the tendon from the bone at this point. In the gluteal region the tendon passes laterally to be inserted into the inner surface of the greater trochanter (Figs 9.2 and 9.3).

As the tendon of the obturator internus passes around the sciatic notch a few muscle fibres arise from the bone of the notch above and below it. These fibres insert into the tendon of the obturator internus. They have been given separate names and are called the **superior and inferior gemellus**. Functionally they can be regarded as part of the obturator internus muscle (Fig. 9.3). The obturator internus is a **lateral rotator** of the hip and is supplied by a branch from the sacral plexus.

Below the obturator internus lies the **quadratus femoris**. This muscle arises from the ischial tuberosity and passes horizontally into the greater trochanter where its insertion produces a raised area called the **quadrate tubercle**. This muscle also is a **lateral rotator** of the hip and is supplied by a nerve from the sacral plexus (Fig. 9.3). There is one more **lateral rotator** to describe. This muscle was mentioned when we studied the medial adductor muscles of the thigh and in fact is supplied by the **obturator nerve**. The **obturator externus** muscle arises from the outer surface of the obturator membrane and the surrounding bone. Its

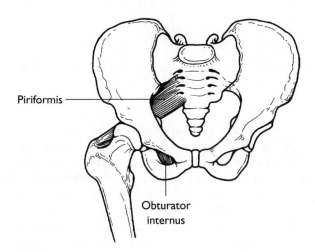

Figure 9.2 Piriformis and obturator internus both arise within the pelvis and pass to the back of the femur behind the hip joint.

tendon sweeps around the back of the capsule of the hip joint to insert into the trochanteric fossa.

Figure 9.4 is a summary diagram of the six small lateral rotators that are found at the back of the hip joint. On to this picture of the deep lateral rotators of the hip we need to add two muscles which, functionally, are stabilizers of the pelvis. These are the **gluteus minimus** and **gluteus medius**. The **gluteus minimus** arises from the lower part of the outer aspect of the iliac blade and inserts into the front of the greater trochanter. It is a 'fan-shaped' muscle (Fig. 9.5). Between it and the greater trochanter, on the deep surface of the muscle, there is a bursa. The gluteus minimus is supplied by the superior gluteal nerve, a branch of the sacral plexus. The **gluteus medius** is also a fan-shaped stabilizer of the pelvis like the minimus, but is a more massive and powerful muscle (Fig. 9.6). It arises from the area of iliac blade between the minimus below and the iliac crest above (between the anterior and posterior gluteal lines). Thus, as it passes down to its insertion into the upper lateral aspect of the greater trochanter, it covers the minimus. It is supplied, like the minimus, by the superior gluteal nerve. The minimus and medius prevent tilting of the pelvis when a foot from the opposite side is raised from the ground, as, for example, during walking (Fig. 9.7). The gluteus minimus and medius are extremely important muscles. They can also abduct the lower limb at the hip joint, but this is not such a common action as stabilization of the pelvis during locomotion.

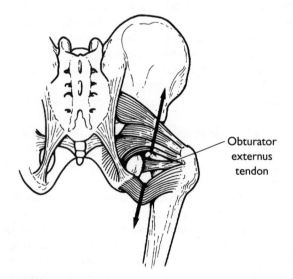

Figure 9.4   When the most posterior lateral rotators are retracted, the obturator externus tendon can be seen running to the trochanteric fossa.

Obturator externus tendon

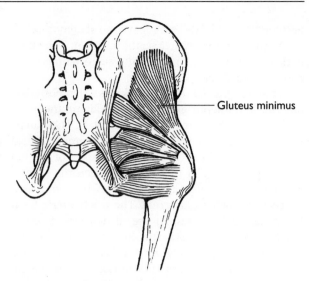

Gluteus minimus

Figure 9.5   Gluteus minimus runs from the anterior gluteal line on the ilium and the bone below this level to the greater trochanter of the femur.

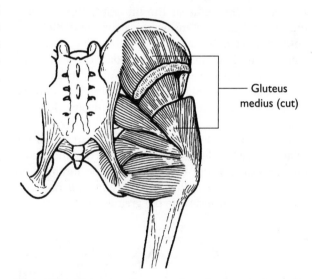

Gluteus medius (cut)

Figure 9.6   Gluteus medius passes from the bone between the posterior and anterior gluteal lines on the ilium to the greater trochanter of the femur.

The function of these muscles can be tested clinically by asking patients to raise each foot from the ground in turn while the pelvis is examined for tilt. If one set of muscles is paralysed, the pelvis falls on the side of the raised foot (Fig. 9.7). The patient is said to have a positive **Trendelenburg sign**. This signifies either a non-functioning gluteus minimus and medius or a hip deformity which is preventing these muscles from working.

A large powerful muscle called the **gluteus max-**

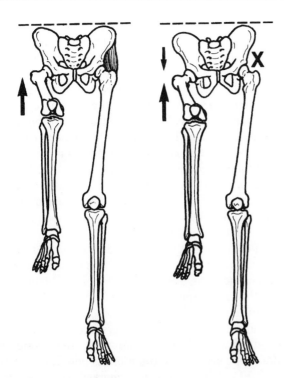

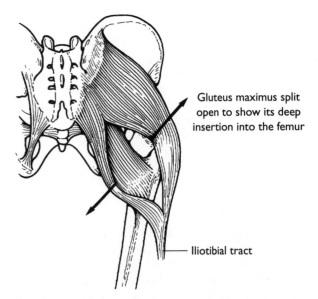

Figure 9.8 Gluteus maximus runs from the most posterior part of the iliac blade (behind the posterior gluteal line) to insert into the gluteal tuberosity of the femur and the iliotibial tract.

Figure 9.7 When one foot is raised off the ground, as when walking, the contralateral gluteus minimus and medius stabilize the pelvis and maintain it in the horizontal plane. When these muscles are ineffective (X) the pelvis falls as the leg is raised.

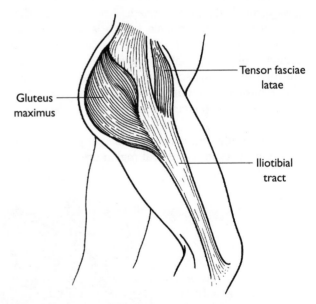

Figure 9.9 The iliotibial tract runs from the tubercle of the iliac crest above, to the side of the lateral condyle of the tibia below.

imus covers both the lateral rotators and the stabilizers of the hip joint. The gluteus maximus is a powerful **extensor** of the hip joint. The gluteus maximus arises from the posterior part of the iliac crest, from the sacrotuberous ligament and from the posterior aspects of the sacrum and coccyx. The coarse muscle fibres pass obliquely, downwards and forwards. Only the lower, deep ones gain attachment to the femur at the **gluteal tuberosity** (Fig. 9.8). The main mass of muscle is superficial and gains insertion into the **iliotibial tract** (Fig. 9.9). The iliotibial tract is a thickening in the deep fascia of the thigh. Above, the iliotibial tract is attached to the tubercle of the iliac crest. The main mass of the tract passes vertically downwards over the lateral side of the knee to insert into the lateral condyle of the tibia. A few fibres in fact pass into the patella. The gluteus maximus is inserted into the tract from behind. In front a small muscle called the **tensor fasciae latae** inserts into the tract. This muscle arises from the iliac crest in front of the tract. The tract therefore serves as a long tendon for the insertions of both the gluteus maximus and the tensor fasciae latae into the lateral condyle of the tibia. In the standing position the iliotibial tract acts as a brace which steadies the pelvis on the femur in the extended position and it also helps to keep the knee joint straight and locked. The rest of the gluteus maximus is a powerful **extensor** of the hip joint. It can straighten the lower limb on the trunk or the trunk on the lower limb. The gluteus maximus is supplied by the **inferior glu-**

teal nerve and the tensor by the **superior gluteal nerve**. There are usually several bursae deep to the gluteus maximus. There is usually a large one between it and the ischial tuberosity. Another is usually seen between the muscle and the greater trochanter and yet one more far laterally between the muscle and the upper part of the vastus lateralis.

Neurovascular structures in the gluteal region

The greater sciatic foramen is the posterior exit from the abdominopelvic cavity. Through it pass the piriformis surrounded by the terminal branches of the sacral plexus. These branches supply motor and sensory innervation to the back of the leg and the buttock. The blood supply to the gluteal region is rich. It is derived from terminal branches of the internal iliac arteries. These too, with their accompanying veins, pass through the greater sciatic foramen. The other great neurovascular bundle, which is also made up of a terminal branch of the sacral plexus and branches of the internal iliac vessels, leaves the pelvis through the greater sciatic foramen as well. But then this neurovascular bundle curls around the ischial spine and enters the perineum through the lesser sciatic foramen.

The muscular branches of the sacral plexus which supply muscles in the gluteal region are the **superior** and **inferior gluteal nerves**, the nerve to the **quadratus femoris** and the nerve to the **obturator internus**. As their names suggest, the superior gluteal nerve leaves the greater sciatic foramen above the piriformis muscle and the inferior gluteal nerve below this muscle (Fig. 9.10). The nerve to the quadratus femoris leaves below the piriformis as well. The nerve to the obturator internus also leaves at the lower border of the piriformis, but then curls around the ischial spine and enters the muscle before it emerges through the lesser sciatic foramen. The cutaneous branch of the sacral plexus seen in this region is the **posterior cutaneous nerve of the thigh**. This carries sensation from skin on the back of the thigh.

By far the largest branch of the lumbar and sacral plexuses is a mixed nerve called the **sciatic nerve**. It contains neurons from the ventral rami of the 4th and 5th lumbar spinal nerves and the first three sacral ventral rami. It emerges at the lower border of the piriformis. At this point it covers over the nerve to the quadratus femoris and has the posterior cutaneous nerve of the thigh on its posterior surface (Fig. 9.11). Its position can be marked on the surface of the buttock midway between the ischial tuberosity and the greater trochanter. From its point of emergence, the sciatic nerve passes down the back of the thigh. At first it is superficial to the lateral rotators. It is enclosed in a condensation of fascia and accompanied by a 'companion artery' which is a small branch of the inferior gluteal artery. While in the buttock, the sciatic nerve is covered by the gluteus

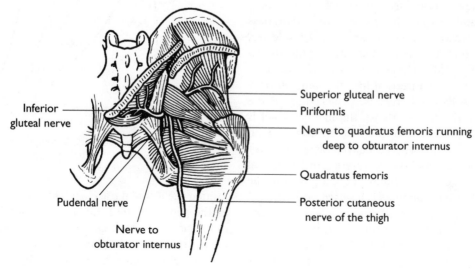

Inferior gluteal nerve

Pudendal nerve

Nerve to obturator internus

Superior gluteal nerve
Piriformis
Nerve to quadratus femoris running deep to obturator internus
Quadratus femoris
Posterior cutaneous nerve of the thigh

Figure 9.10 Piriformis is the key to understanding the gluteal region. The superior gluteal nerves emerge from its upper border. The inferior gluteal nerves emerge from its lower border.

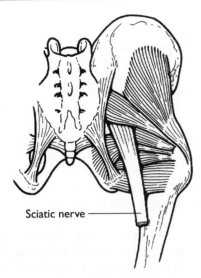

Figure 9.11   The sciatic nerve covers the posterior cutaneous nerve of the thigh and the exposed part of the nerve to quadratus femoris, as it emerges below the lower border of piriformis.

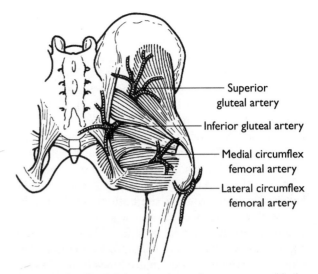

Figure 9.12   The inferior gluteal vessels anastomose with the circumflex vessels of the profunda femoris and the uppermost perforators to form the cruciate anastomosis behind the hip joint.

maximus. It then enters the back of the thigh by passing on to the posterior surface of the adductor magnus. At some point in its course, the sciatic nerve divides into two branches. These are the **common peroneal** and **tibial nerves**. This division usually takes place in the back of the thigh, but sometimes it is found in the gluteal region or even in the pelvis. If the division takes place in the pelvis the common peroneal nerve usually pierces the piriformis muscle as it enters the gluteal region.

The gluteal region is richly supplied with blood since there is such a large mass of musculature here. It is worth noting, though, that there is no equivalent to the femoral artery in the anterior compartment of the thigh, accompanying the sciatic nerve out of the pelvis posteriorly. The profunda femoris is the artery that supplies the back of the thigh. The **superior gluteal artery** is a branch of the internal iliac artery and this large vessel enters the region in company with the superior gluteal nerve. Similarly, the **inferior gluteal artery**, also a branch of the internal iliac, enters with the inferior gluteal nerve. Great veins accompany these big neurovascular bundles and they drain into the internal iliac veins. However, some of the blood supply from the region comes up through branches of the lateral and medial circumflex arteries (Fig. 9.12). The anastomosis of these circumflex vessels with the inferior gluteal vessels above and the perforators below forms the so-called **cruciate anastomosis**. We have seen that the neurovascular bundle,

destined to supply the perineum, leaves the pelvis through the greater sciatic foramen and then immediately enters the perineum through the lesser sciatic foramen. It is therefore seen passing for a short distance through the region we are studying now (Fig. 9.10). The **pudendal nerve** curls around the sacrospinous ligament. The internal pudendal artery accompanied by its venae comitantes curls around near the tip of the spine of the ischium.

Applied anatomy of the gluteal region

This is a good time to reconsider the femoral artery and the profunda femoris artery in the thigh. There is a rich anastomosis between the profunda femoris artery and the vessels of the cruciate anastomosis posteriorly. When there is damage to the femoral artery high up, proximal to the origin of the profunda, blood from these rich anastomoses with the profunda may flow into it 'the wrong way' and so perfuse the leg. Much more serious is obstruction or damage to the femoral artery distal to the profunda femoris artery. In this situation gangrene of the foot and tissue death from ischaemia is likely since no blood can reach the leg via any anastomosis with the profunda.

By far the most important structure in the gluteal

region is the sciatic nerve. This is one of the few nerves in the body where a neuronal component needs to be learned. It is made up of neurons from the ventral rami of L4 and L5, and S1, 2 and 3. To understand the importance of this composition consider the anatomy of herniated intervertebral discs. This most frequently occurs between the 4th and 5th lumbar or 5th lumbar vertebrae and the sacrum. Therefore one of the commonest complaints following disc trouble is **sciatica**, or pain somewhere along the course of the sciatic nerve. This can occasionally be localized pain felt only in the buttock but it usually passes down the back of the leg. It may also be accompanied by anaesthesia of the skin in the lower leg if sensory neurons are damaged by the disc. The sciatic nerve may also be injured locally in the buttock. Intramuscular injections are frequently given into the mass of the gluteal musculature (Fig. 9.13). This is easily done by drawing two lines on the buttock to divide it into four equal quadrants. An injection should be given deeply into the upper and outer quadrant. This avoids injury to the sciatic nerve. A safer place for intramuscular injections is into the vastus lateralis mass in the thigh.

The hip joint

The proximal parts of the thigh musculature and the gluteal region surround the hip joint. The **hip joint** is, like the shoulder joint, a ball and socket type of synovial joint but although the lower limb needs to be mobile it must also be weight bearing and therefore

stable. Thus it might be said that the hip joint gives up a little mobility for stability. The **articular surfaces** of the hip joint are the **head of the femur** and the **acetabulum** of the innominate bone or pelvis. The head of the femur is spherical and covered, in life, with articular cartilage (Fig. 9.14). The circumference of the femoral neck is less than that of the head. This is in contrast to the thick anatomical neck of the humerus. The femoral neck is therefore more susceptible to fracture. In the centre of the head there is a small pit. Here, several small holes may be seen on a dry specimen, through which nutrient arteries enter to supply the bone.

The acetabulum is formed from parts of the ilium, pubis and ischium. Ossification is completed here soon after puberty. The acetabulum is deepened considerably by a fibrocartilaginous rim called the **labrum acetabulare** (Fig. 9.15). However, near the obturator foramen, the wall of the acetabulum is deficient, forming the **acetabular notch**. The circle of the labrum is completed in this region by a fibrous bridge which spans the acetabular notch. This is called the **transverse ligament**. In life, a branch of the obturator artery supplies the femoral head by passing through the acetabular notch. In its journey beneath the transverse ligament to the pit in the femoral head it is surrounded by a condensation of fibrous tissue called the **ligament of the head of the femur**. This 'ligament' does not, however, function to strengthen the hip joint.

The fibrous capsule of the hip joint is very strong and is responsible for much of the strength of the joint. Its fibres pass from the circumference of the acetabulum to the femoral neck. Some fibres, how-

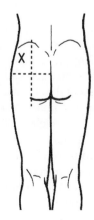

Figure 9.13 Intramuscular injections into the buttock are given into the upper outer quadrant to avoid damage to the sciatic nerve.

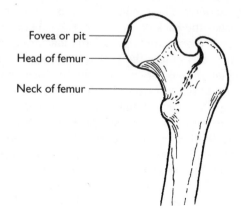

Fovea or pit ———
Head of femur ———
Neck of femur ———

Figure 9.14 The spherical head of the femur is set on the narrower neck at an oblique angle to the shaft of the femur.

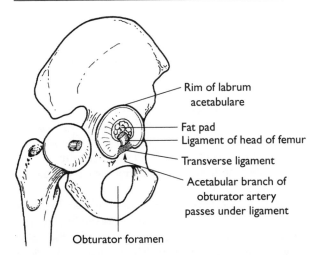

Rim of labrum
acetabulare

Fat pad

Ligament of head of femur

Transverse ligament

Acetabular branch of
obturator artery
passes under ligament

Obturator foramen

Figure 9.15 The transverse ligament spans the acetabular notch. The fibrocartilaginous labrum acetabulare greatly deepens the acetabulum.

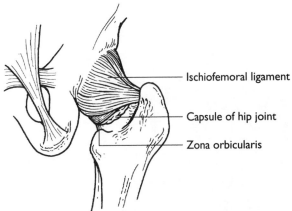

Ischiofemoral ligament

Capsule of hip joint

Zona orbicularis

Figure 9.17 The ischiofemoral ligament behind the hip joint capsule runs short of the joint capsule, which can be seen protruding beneath it. The innermost fibres of the ligaments surrounding the capsule run in a circular fashion in the zona orbicularis around the neck of the femur.

ever, pass in a circular fashion around the capsule to form a band called the **zona orbicularis**. Various parts of the capsule are strengthened to form ligament. The front of the capsule is greatly strengthened as the **iliofemoral ligament** (Fig. 9.16). Proximally, the fibres of this ligament gain attachment to the anterior inferior iliac spine and the labrum. Distally they insert into the intertrochanteric line on the front of the femur. The central part of the ligament is thin so that the ligament gives the impression of an inverted 'Y'-shaped thickening. It is one of the strongest ligaments in the body.

The lower part of the capsule is strengthened as a thick **pubofemoral ligament**. The fibres that constitute this ligament pass between the pubic bone and the lowermost part of the intertrochanteric line. Behind, the joint the capsule is not so strong but there is a thickening in this region which is called the **ischiofemoral ligament**. These fibres pass between the ischium just below the acetabulum and the neck of the femur (Fig. 9.17). Some capsular fibres run along the neck of the femur from the capsular attachment as far as the head. These are the **retinacular fibres** (Fig. 9.18). Like the ligament of the head of the femur, they give support to blood vessels. The blood supply to the femoral head and neck is important and this is a convenient time to review it.

Most of the blood comes from branches of the

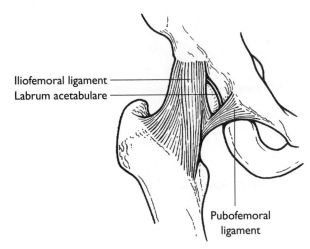

Iliofemoral ligament

Labrum acetabulare

Pubofemoral
ligament

Figure 9.16 The strong iliofemoral ligament runs from the anterior inferior iliac spine to the intertrochanteric line on the femur. It prevents the trunk extending backwards at the hip joint when standing.

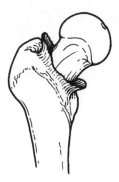

Figure 9.18 Some capsular fibres run as far as the head of the femur and give support for blood vessels. These are the retinacular fibres.

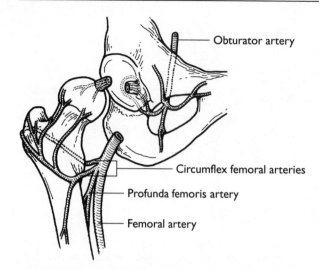

Figure 9.19 Blood to the bone of the head and neck of the femur comes partly from the superior gluteal artery (not shown) but mostly from the circumflex femoral arteries, obturator artery and cruciate anastomosis posteriorly (after Hollinshead, WH (1982) *Anatomy for Surgeons*, 3rd edn. Philadelphia: Harper and Row).

medial and **lateral circumflex arteries** but there is also a contribution from the **superior gluteal artery**. These branches pass along the femoral neck, protected by the retinacular fibres, and enter the bone at various points around the neck (Fig. 9.19). There is also some blood supply from the **artery of the ligament of the head of the femur**. This is a branch of the obturator artery which passes through the acetabular notch, deep to the transverse ligament. The artery is protected by the ligament of the head of the femur as it passes to the femoral head where it enters the bone. At this point it produces a pit and a foramen which can be clearly seen in the head of the femur.

Synovial membrane lines the non-articular parts of the hip joint. It lines the capsule, covers a fat pad in the central deep part of the acetabulum, and gives a tubular investment to the ligament of the head of the femur. The strength and stability of the hip joint derive from several factors. These include the deep cup-shaped labrum which holds the femoral head in the acetabulum, the ligaments that surround the joint, and the surrounding muscle mass that pulls the head of the femur into the acetabulum. The oblique direction of the neck of the femur also helps since there is no tendency to dislocate during standing but, rather, force is transmitted in towards the acetabulum.

The femur can flex, extend, abduct and adduct at the hip joint. A combination of all these movements is called circumduction. The femur can also rotate in

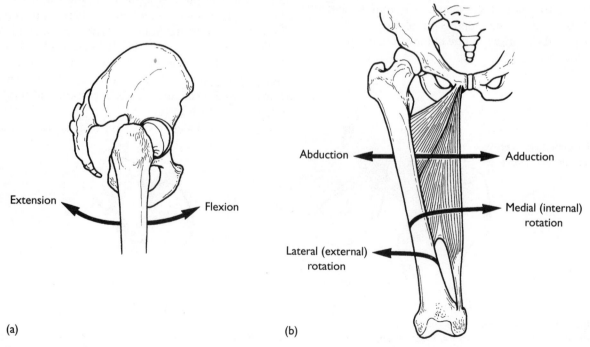

(a)   (b)

Figure 9.20 (a) Extension and flexion, (b) abduction and adduction all occur at the hip joint. Rotation in the long axis of the femur produces either medial or lateral rotation of the thigh.

its long axis to produce the movements of **lateral** and **medial rotation** (Fig. 9.20). In full flexion, the knee can be brought up to touch the abdomen. This movement is produced by the iliopsoas muscle. Extension of the hip joint is checked by the iliofemoral ligament. Extension is brought about mainly by the gluteus maximus. Abduction is not a movement commonly employed, by most of us at least, but the gluteus medius and minimus act as powerful pelvic stabilizers during walking or when standing on one leg. The adductors make up a powerful mass on the medial side of the thigh and the hip may be adducted so that the one leg crosses over the other. In fact the adductor muscles act to pull the trunk over the stance leg during walking more often than they do to cross the leg. Lateral rotation of the femur is produced by the small lateral rotators at the back of the hip joint. Medial rotation is limited by the spiralling of the fibres of the capsule during this movement. The chief muscles involved in this movement are the anterior fibres of the pelvic stabilizers, that is the gluteus medius and minimus. Medial rotation is also brought about by the iliopsoas when the thigh is flexed. Tensor fasciae latae also tends to medially rotate the thigh as well. Place your hand over your hip and rotate your femur medially. You will feel the contraction of the gluteal fibres and the tensor fasciae latae. Some of the adductor group may also be active during medial rotation.

The hip joint, like the shoulder joint, is surrounded by muscle. There are, however, also important neurovascular relationships around the joint. In front the most important of these is the femoral artery and femoral nerve. Behind the joint it is the sciatic nerve that is most important to remember.

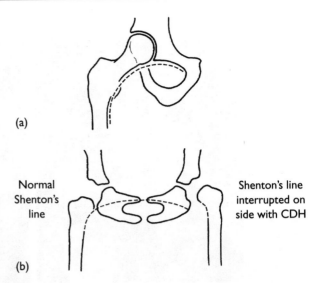

(a)

Normal
Shenton's
line

Shenton's line
interrupted on
side with CDH

(b)

Figure 9.21 (a) Shenton's line is a smooth, uninterrupted curved line that runs from the neck of the femur into the upper border of the obturator foramen on a radiograph of the hip joint. (b) In this case of CDH, in an infant in whom the epiphysis has not yet appeared, Shenton's line is interrupted.

abnormal joint by drawing **Shenton's lines** on a radiograph (Fig. 9.21). This line runs in continuity from the upper border of the obturator foramen to the lower border of the neck of the femur. It is normally a direct, uninterrupted, curved line. In CDH the line is broken. The epiphysis for the head of the femur has usually appeared on a radiograph by the time the child is 1 year old. In CDH it is usually small and late to appear. When the epiphysis appears, however, and when a child is examined at the age of about 9 months onwards, CDH may be determined on a radiograph by drawing **Perkin's lines** (Fig. 9.22). One line

Applied anatomy of the hip joint

The hip is immensely important clinically. The hip joint and proximal end of the femur are frequently involved in injuries and bone diseases. At birth some infants are born with congenital dislocation of one or other hip joints. The condition is usually called CDH. This needs to be detected at birth by abducting the flexed leg of the baby. In cases of CDH. there is an audible 'click' as the head of the femur slips back into its socket. The head of the femur is cartilaginous during the first year of life and therefore cannot be seen on radiographs. However, it is possible to detect an

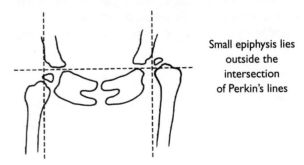

Small epiphysis lies
outside the
intersection
of Perkin's lines

Figure 9.22 Perkin's lines run horizontally through the centres of the epiphyses of the femoral heads in one plane, and vertically (perpendicular to horizontal line) at the outer lips of the acetabulae.

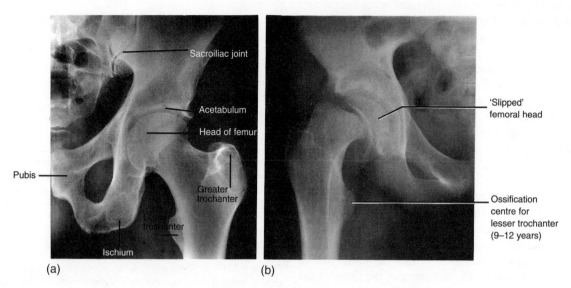

(a)   (b)

Figure 9.23   Radiograph of a normal adult hip joint (a) compared with that of a boy with a slipped epiphysis across the growth disc (b). A few key landmarks are indicated on the adult hip.

is drawn horizontally through the centres of the acetabulae and then two lines are drawn vertically at the outer lip of the acetabulum. Normally, the epiphysis for the head of the femur lies *below* the horizontal and *internal* to the vertical line. In CDH the head is displaced outwards and upwards (Fig. 9.22).

Occasionally, between the ages of 5 and 10 years, there is a bony degeneration of the head of the femur. This is known as **Perthes' disease**. It may be due to trauma which interferes with the blood supply to the growing head. The condition typically runs a course of degeneration and then recovery. Treatment therefore consists of holding the hip in a rested position and then awaiting recovery.

Children between the ages of 10 and 15 years who fall and injure their hip joints, before the head of the femur has fused with the shaft, occasionally fracture the femur across the growth disc, a so-called **slipped epiphysis** (Fig. 9.23). If not replaced, union results in deformity of the femoral head and neck, and later osteoarthritis.

In old age, fractures tend to dominate in the region of the femoral neck or intertrochanteric regions. Occasionally a fracture across the femoral neck can cut off the blood supply to the head of the femur such that the bone dies and becomes necrotic. Many fractures of the femoral neck and intertrochanteric regions are fixed by metal pins or plates. Radiographs of the hip joint in middle-aged and elderly people often show the 'tell-tale' signs of osteoarthritic disease. These include loss of joint space (loss of articular cartilage), irregular, spiked bony margins called osteophytes and some change in bone density near the articulation.

chapter

10

The Back of the Thigh, Popliteal Fossa and Knee Joint

The back of the thigh lies distal to the gluteal area and the hip joint. The compartment at the back of the thigh is occupied by the **flexor muscles of the knee** and all of these arise from the **ischial tuberosity**. They pass down to insert into the **medial, posterior** and **lateral** aspects of the knee. They are all supplied by the **sciatic nerve**. There are three muscles in this region that we need to study first. They are called the **semitendinosus**, the **semimembranosus** and the **biceps**. They all arise from the ischial tuberosity and pass down the back of the thigh as a fleshy mass in the gutter formed by the posterior surface of the adductor magnus and the lateral intermuscular septum (Fig. 10.1).

The **semitendinosus** passes to its insertion at the medial side of the knee. Look carefully at this insertion. It lies behind the insertions of two other muscles that have already been studied. These are the tendons of the **gracilis** and **sartorius** (Figs 10.2 and 10.3). Both of these tendons insert into the medial aspect of the tibia just below the knee. The semitendinosus inserts into the tibia just behind the gracilis (Fig. 10.3). The muscle is supplied by the **tibial part** of the **sciatic nerve**. Its main action is to flex the knee joint, but since it arises from the ischium it also has a weak extending action on the hip.

The **semimembranosus** arises from the ischial tuberosity and passes down with the semitendinosus muscle. Its insertion is extensive since the tendon fans out as several **aponeurotic expansions** at the back of the knee joint. The tendon inserts into the back of the medial condyle of the tibia and the expansions blend with the capsule of the knee joint and attach to the **soleal line** on the back of the tibia (Fig. 10.4). The

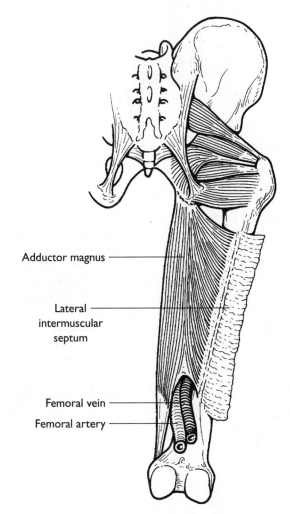

Figure 10.1 Adductor magnus, the adductor hiatus and the lateral intermuscular septum seen from behind.

Adductor magnus

Lateral intermuscular septum

Femoral vein

Femoral artery

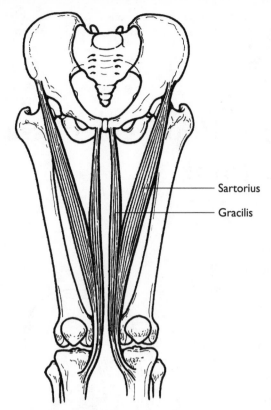

Figure 10.2 Note how the tendons of sartorius and gracilis run to the medial aspect of the medial tibial condyle.

thickening produced by the expansion at the back of the knee joint capsule is called the **posterior oblique ligament** and the expansion which gains attachment to the soleal line covers a small muscle in the region called the **popliteus**. The muscle is supplied in the same way as the semitendinosus by the tibial part of the sciatic nerve, and it has the same actions.

The **biceps femoris** arises from the ischial tuberosity and passes down to the lateral aspect of the knee (Figs 10.4 and 10.5). The muscle, as its name implies, arises by means of two bellies. It is the **long head** that arises from the tuberosity, the **short head** arising from the lower part of the linea aspera of the femur. The tendon of the combined muscle inserts into the **head of the fibula**.

The long head of the biceps is supplied by the **tibial part** of the sciatic nerve but the short head gains its supply from the **common peroneal part** of the sciatic nerve. Notice that the lower ends of the three muscles, **semitendinosus**, **semimembranosus** and **biceps**, make an inverted 'V' shape. The semimembranosus and the

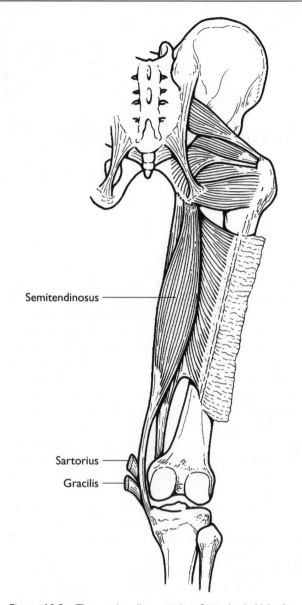

Figure 10.3 The semitendinosus arises from the ischial tuberosity and passes to its insertion at the medial tibial condyle, behind those of gracilis and sartorius.

semitendinosus muscles form one limb of the 'V' and the biceps the other (Fig. 10.6).

The muscle at the back of the lower leg arises as two heads in another 'V' shape (but the 'right way up' this time). This muscle is called the **gastrocnemius**. The two heads arise from the back of the femoral condyles. Thus, if the muscles are separated, as in Figure 10.6, they form a diamond-shaped hollow behind the knee. This hollow is called the **popliteal fossa**. After separating the muscles that bound

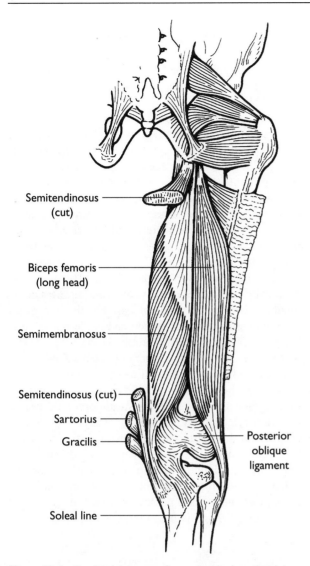

Semitendinosus (cut)

Biceps femoris (long head)

Semimembranosus

Semitendinosus (cut)

Sartorius

Gracilis

Posterior oblique ligament

Soleal line

Figure 10.4 Semimembranosus fans out at its insertion into a posterior oblique ligament, behind the capsule of the knee joint, and an expansion overlying the popliteus which then runs to the soleal line on the tibia.

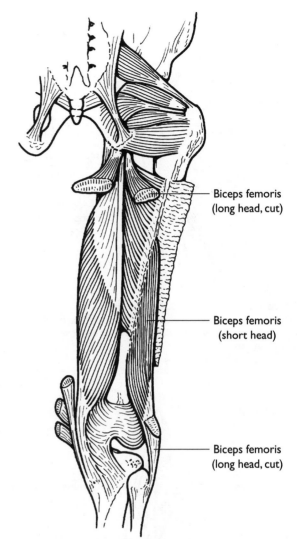

Biceps femoris (long head, cut)

Biceps femoris (short head)

Biceps femoris (long head, cut)

Figure 10.5 The long and short heads of biceps femoris converge and insert on to the head of the fibula.

the popliteal fossa, the depths of this hollow may be examined. This is the posterior aspect of the knee joint. In this region the capsule is strengthened by an expansion of the semimembranosus called the posterior oblique ligament. The expansion that covers the popliteus muscle can also be seen. The fossa contains a fair amount of fat.

The nerve of the back of the thigh is the **sciatic nerve.** We have already traced it from the greater sciatic foramen over the surface of the small lateral rotators of the hip joint. In this part of its course it is covered by the great gluteal muscle mass. The nerve continues its course down through the posterior compartment covered by the biceps. At some variable point in its course it divides into **tibial** and **common peroneal nerves.** The tibial nerve enters the popliteal fossa at the upper angle. It is the most superficial structure in the fossa. It disappears from view at the lower angle of the fossa. While in the back of the thigh and popliteal fossa, the tibial nerve supplies the semimembranosus, tendinosus and long head of the biceps. It gives articular twigs to the knee joint and a small cutaneous nerve leaves it and descends in the subcutaneous fat down the midline of the back of the leg. This nerve is called the **sural** branch (Fig. 10.7).

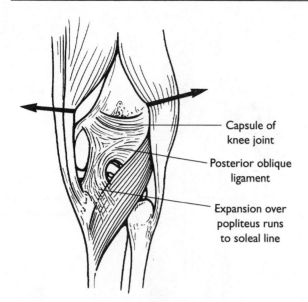

Figure 10.6 Semitendinosus, semimembranosus and biceps femoris form an inverted 'V' shape in the popliteal region which when retracted reveals the deep tendinous expansions of semimembranosus.

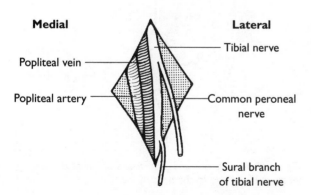

Figure 10.7 Within the popliteal fossa, the deepest structure is the popliteal artery and the most superficial the tibial nerve.

The **common peroneal nerve** enters the fossa with the tibial nerve at the upper angle. But it then leaves the fossa by curling over the lateral edge of the fossa at its lateral angle. In this way it reaches the neck of the fibula and can be rolled by a finger against the bone in this region. The common peroneal nerve divides into **superficial** and **deep peroneal nerves**. It supplies the short head of the biceps in the thigh and also gives articular and cutaneous twigs.

Blood supply to the back of the thigh

The blood supply to the back of the thigh comes from the perforating branches of the profunda femoris (Fig. 8.21). In the lower part of the thigh, however, the femoral artery passes through the hole in the adductor magnus and enters the popliteal fossa. Once it has passed into the fossa it is renamed the **popliteal artery**. The artery is the deepest structure in the fossa, lying in contact with the back of the knee joint capsule and fascial sheets of the semimembranosus. It terminates at the lower angle of the fossa by dividing into the **anterior** and **posterior tibial arteries**. While in the fossa the artery gives several 'genicular branches' to the knee joint (Fig. 10.8). The accompanying vein for the artery is the **popliteal vein**. This is formed distally by confluence of the venae commitantes of the tibial arteries. In the popliteal fossa it is the intermediate member of the neurovascular bundle made up of the popliteal artery, vein and tibial nerve (Fig. 10.8). It receives the **short saphenous vein**. This vessel drains blood from the lateral aspect of the ankle and runs up in the subcutaneous fat in the midline at the back of the leg (along with the sural nerve). On reaching the back of the knee it dips deeply, piercing the deep fascia, and enters the popliteal vein. The popliteal vein leaves the fossa by passing through the hiatus in the adductor magnus along with the artery. It is renamed on the front of the thigh and becomes the **femoral vein**. As it passes through the opening in the adductor magnus it lies lateral to the artery.

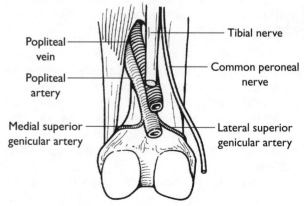

Figure 10.8 The tibial nerve joins the popliteal vessels as they emerge through the adductor hiatus.

The deep fascial coverings of the thigh

The thigh is surrounded by a dense sleeve of **deep fascia** which is given the name of the **fascia lata**. Its attachment around the root of the limb may be traced from the iliac crest along the inguinal ligament to the pubic arch and then to the ischial tuberosity (Fig. 10.9). Posteriorly it is continuous with the deep fascia over the gluteal muscles, and by this means it is attached to the sacrum, coccyx and sacrotuberous ligaments. Just below the medial end of the inguinal ligament the deep fascia presents an oval defect. This is the **saphenous opening** which is plugged with a little areolar tissue called the cribriform fascia (Fig. 8.23). The outer edge of the saphenous opening is sharp and is called the **falciform margin**. The medial edge blends with the fascia of the underlying muscles. The **great saphenous vein** pierces this opening when it dips deeply into the thigh to enter the femoral vein. A few lymphatics also pierce the cribriform fascia.

Distally, the fascia lata is attached to the patella, to the margins of the tibia and to the head of the fibula (Fig. 10.10). Behind the knee joint it covers the popliteal fossa and is here called the **popliteal fascia**. The **small saphenous vein** pierces the popliteal fascia to enter the popliteal vein. On the lateral side of the thigh the fascia lata is thickened to form a strong strap-like band which extends from the iliac crest above to the lateral aspect of the tibia below. This is the **iliotibial tract**. The tract with its muscles, the ten-

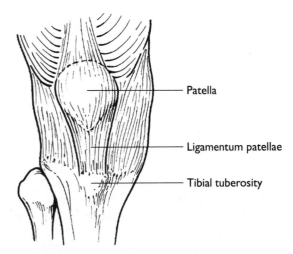

Figure 10.10 Distally, the fascia lata extends down to the patella and knee in front. It covers the popliteal fossa posteriorly.

sor fasciae latae and the gluteus maximus, has an important steadying influence on the hip and knee joints.

The deep fascia of the thigh is covered by an outer sleeve of **subcutaneous fat** (Fig. 10.11). In the proximal inch or two on the front of the thigh this fatty layer has the same pattern as that of the lower anterior abdominal wall, scrotal and perineal fatty

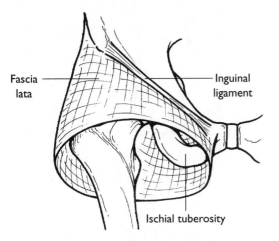

Figure 10.9 The deep fascia of the thigh is called the fascia lata. Its attachment runs around the inguinal ligament, pubic arch, ischial tuberosity and over the iliac crest.

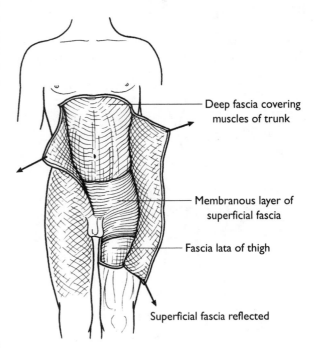

Figure 10.11 The layers of superficial fascia and their relationship to the deep fascia lata of the thigh.

layers. The peculiar pattern found in these regions is due to the deepest layer of fat being condensed into a **membranous layer**. This membranous condensation of the deep subcutaneous fat is found only in these regions, and distally it soon fuses with the fascia lata of the thigh. It has one very important clinical application. Following rupture of the urethra in the perineum, urine may track between the deep fascia and this membrane (see Volume 3). The membranous condensation of superficial fascia directs the urine up over the anterior abdominal wall in this tissue plane. It cannot spread down the thigh because of the attachment of the membranous layer to the fascia lata. Indeed the membranous condensation of the subcutaneous fat can be thought of as looking very much like a kangaroo's pouch. It certainly behaves like that following rupture of the urethra (Fig. 10.11).

The knee joint

The knee joint is a synovial joint of the hinge variety. This means that the only movements at the joint would be **flexion** and **extension** (Fig. 10.12). However, such a simple statement must be modified since a small amount of rotation between the femur and tibia is possible, especially in the flexed position of the joint.

The articular surfaces of the joint consist of the condyles of the femur and the flat upper surfaces of the

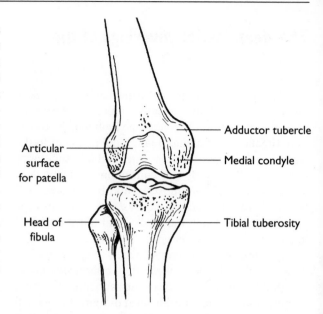

Figure 10.13   Bony landmarks on the front of the femur, fibula and tibia at the knee joint.

tibial condyles (Figs 10.13 and 10.14). The lateral and medial condyles of the femur and the tibial plateaux are covered with articular cartilage. The tibial condyles are separated from each other by a midline ridge called the **intercondylar eminence**. Lying on the

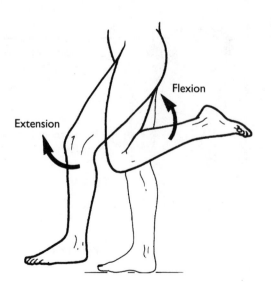

Figure 10.12   Flexion and extension taking place at the knee joint.

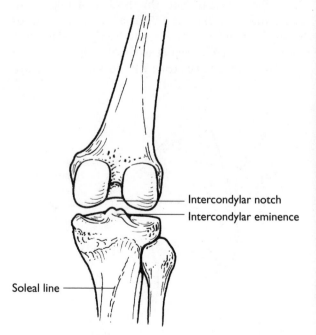

Figure 10.14   Bony landmarks on the back of the femur and tibia at the knee joint.

flat tibial condyles are two 'C'-shaped fibrocartilages called the **lateral** and **medial menisci**. The pointed ends of these structures point towards the intercondylar eminence and are called the **horns** of the menisci (Fig. 10.15). The menisci are attached to the tibial surface by fibrous tissue both at the horns and at their outer crescentic margins. The inner edges of the menisci are thin and so they present a saucer-shaped articular surface for each femoral condyle rather than two flat surfaces. The medial meniscus is oval in shape whereas the lateral meniscus is circular. The two menisci are united anteriorly by a fibrous band called the **transverse ligament**. In spite of the attachments of the menisci to the tibia they do have a certain degree of mobility on the tibial surfaces. They are able to 'fill in' the joint space during movements. The transverse ligament prevents the menisci moving apart and also ensures that there is some degree of interaction between the two menisci.

The fibrous capsule of the knee joint is incomplete. In front it is largely replaced by the tendon of the quadriceps, the patella and the ligamentum patellae (Fig. 10.16). The **patella** articulates with the front of the femur at all times, and never with the tibia. Its deep surface is covered with cartilage and this articulates with cartilage found in the midline on the femur and with a crescentic area of cartilage on the medial femoral condyle (Fig. 10.16). A faint line demarcates these two areas on the articular surface of the patella. The articular cartilage of the patella is also faintly divided by horizontal lines into an upper, a middle and

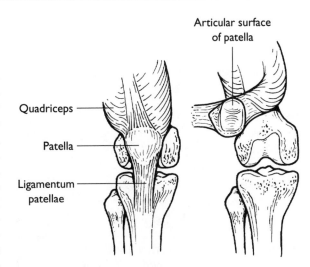

Figure 10.16 In front, the tough capsule of the knee joint is largely replaced by the patella, the tendon of the quadriceps and the ligamentum patellae.

a lower facet. When the knee is flexed it is the upper facet that is in contact with the femur and then, as the knee extends, the other patella facets slide onto the femoral surface.

On either side of the extensor apparatus (quadriceps, patella and ligamentum patellae) the capsule is thin. It extends from the edges of the femoral condyles above to the front of the tibia. Here the capsule is not far beneath the skin, but is strengthened by fascia lata and by fibrous expansions from the vastus lateralis and medialis. These strengthening

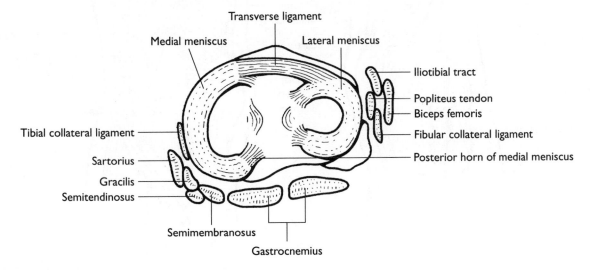

Figure 10.15 Superior view of the proximal tibia showing the menisci, their horns, and the positions of associated muscles and ligaments that are related to the knee joint.

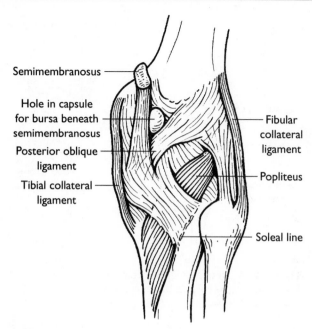

Semimembranosus

Hole in capsule for bursa beneath semimembranosus

Posterior oblique ligament

Tibial collateral ligament

Fibular collateral ligament

Popliteus

Soleal line

Figure 10.17 Posteriorly, the capsule of the knee joint is strengthened by the posterior oblique ligament of the semimembranosus expansion. There are deficiencies in the posterior capsule through which bursae protrude beneath the semimembranosus and beneath the medial head of gastrocnemius.

layers are called the **patella retinacula**. At the back of the joint the capsule stretches from the edges of the femoral condyles to the tibia. It is, however, strengthened by the **posterior oblique ligament** of the knee joint. You will recall that this ligament is one of the expansions of the semimembranosus insertion (Fig. 10.17).

As in all hinge joints, the knee joint capsule is very strong at the sides. The knee joint capsule is strengthened by strong **fibular** and **tibial collateral ligaments**. On the lateral side of the joint there is a strong fibrous band extending from the femur to the head of the fibula (Fig. 10.18). This is the fibular collateral ligament. At its lower insertion it splits the tendon of biceps. The tibial collateral ligament is a flat triangular sheet of fibrous tissue. From its origin at the adductor tubercle of the femur its fibres stretch to the tibia, fanning out as they do so. Some of the deep fibres can be traced through the capsule into the side of the medial meniscus. This attachment of the tibial collateral ligament to the meniscus makes the medial meniscus a little less mobile than the lateral one. A bursa usually separates the three medial tendons (sartorius, gracilis and semitendinosus) from the tibial collateral ligament.

The knee joint is unlike most other joints in that it has two very strong ligaments within the joint itself.

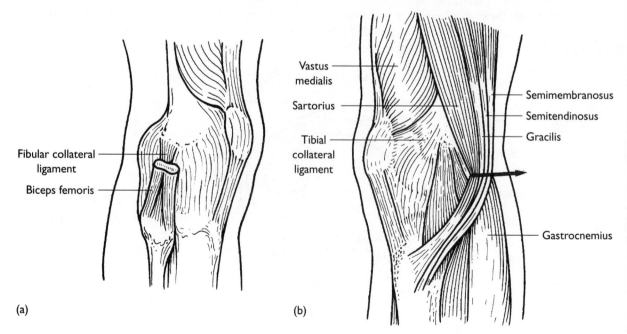

Fibular collateral ligament

Biceps femoris

Vastus medialis

Sartorius

Tibial collateral ligament

Semimembranosus

Semitendinosus

Gracilis

Gastrocnemius

(a)

(b)

Figure 10.18 (a) The round cord-like fibular collateral ligament divides the biceps femoris tendon at the head of the fibula. (b) The medial tibial collateral ligament is flat and triangular and is also attached to the medial meniscus.

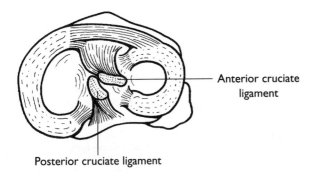

— Anterior cruciate ligament

Posterior cruciate ligament

Figure 10.19 As they twist past each other, the cruciate ligaments cross over to the inner surfaces of the femoral condyles.

These are called the **cruciate ligaments**. They arise from the intercondylar region of the tibia and are named according to their tibial origin. The **anterior cruciate** ligament therefore arises from the anterior part of the intercondylar region, and the **posterior cruciate** ligament from the posterior part. As they pass to their femoral attachments they twist past each other and cross over, inserting into the inner surfaces of the femoral condyles (Fig. 10.19). It can be imagined, therefore, how they are able to prevent the femoral and tibial surfaces slipping anteroposteriorly relative to each other. The **posterior ligament** prevents slipping of the femur *forwards* on the tibia, for example when weight bearing on a flexed knee (Fig. 10.20). The **anterior ligament** prevents slipping during such

movements as extension of the knee, as when walking or kicking a ball (Fig. 10.20). However, on looking at the cruciate ligaments more carefully, you will note that they do not cross each other in the sagittal plane but rather the anterior veers to insert into the **lateral femoral condyle** and the posterior into the **medial femoral condyle** (Fig. 10.19). They therefore also function to prevent excess rotation between the femur and tibia.

The cruciate ligaments help not only to maintain the anteroposterior stability of the knee but also to prevent rotational strains. They are extremely thick and strong. In some knees one or two fibrous strands will be found passing from the back of the lateral meniscus to the posterior cruciate ligament and femoral condyle. These are named the **meniscofemoral ligaments**.

The synovial membrane of the knee joint lines all the inner surfaces of the knee joint except those covered with articular cartilage. This means the inside of the capsule, the cruciate ligaments and the pad of fat that is found at the front of the joint. This pad is called the **infrapatellar fat pad**. The cruciate ligaments are covered on all sides except posteriorly where they are bare (Fig. 10.21). There are several important bursae around the knee joint. Some of these are simply balloons of synovial membrane which bulge out through holes in the capsule. This

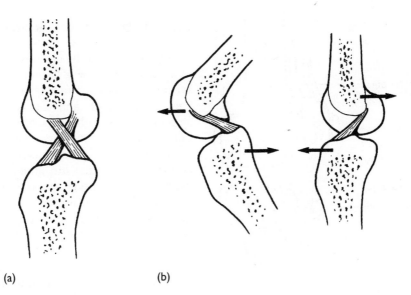

(a)   (b)

Figure 10.20 The cruciate ligaments limit rotational strains at the knee. The posterior cruciate ligament prevents slipping of the femur forwards on the tibia, particularly on a flexed knee. The anterior cruciate ligament prevents posterior displacement of the femur on an extended knee.

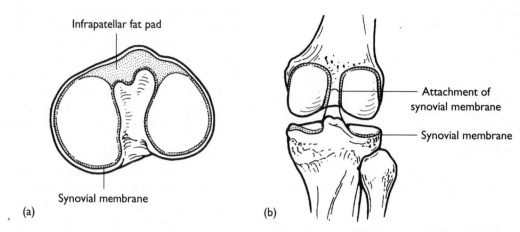

Infrapatellar fat pad

Attachment of
synovial membrane

Synovial membrane

Synovial membrane

(a)   (b)

Figure 10.21   For the most part, the synovial membrane within the knee joint follows the attachment and contours of the joint capsule. However, it runs free of the capsule in between the femoral condyles and in front of the cruciate ligaments.

type of bursa is therefore continuous with the synovial cavity of the joint. Others are separate synovial 'balloons' positioned at places prone to frictional rubbing such as around the tendons crossing the joint (Figs 10.22 and 10.17). The synovial membrane of the knee is continuous above with a large **suprapatellar bursa**. This extends up over the surface of the femur to a level *above* the patella. In conditions in which there is accumulation of synovial fluid in the knee this can often be seen as a fullness above the patella. A few muscular fibres of the vastus intermedius insert into the upper limit of the bursa. (They are often given a special name, the **articularis genu**.) These help to prevent pinching of the bursa into the knee joint during movement. The synovial membrane of the knee is also continuous with a bursa which bulges out through a hole in the posterior capsule (Fig. 10.17). This bursa extends deep to the semimembranosus and to the medial head of gastrocnemius.

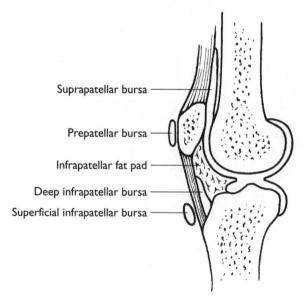

Suprapatellar bursa

Prepatellar bursa

Infrapatellar fat pad

Deep infrapatellar bursa

Superficial infrapatellar bursa

Figure 10.22   The large suprapatellar bursa is continuous with the capsule of the knee joint. Other bursae are separate balloons of synovial fluid positioned between points prone to friction.

Movements of the knee

Being a hinge joint the obvious movements occurring at the knee are those of flexion and extension. Flexion is complete when the calf comes into contact with the back of the thigh and extension when the leg is straight. At first sight the shapes of the joint surfaces of the femur and tibia do not seem to be well designed for a hinge type of movement. However, it is the strong ligaments that surround the knee and the cruciate ligaments inside the knee which ensure that only movements of flexion and extension can take place. None the less, we need to study the small but important rotatory movements that can take place in the knee joint. Place a finger on one of your tibial tuberosities and then, with your knee flexed to a right angle, move your foot so that it first points outwards and then inwards. You will feel a slight rotatory movement of the tibia when these movements are performed. However, the most important rotation at the knee takes place just as the knee joint is reaching full extension. At this last moment in the straightening of the knee there is a slight *medial rotation* of the femur on the tibia. This happens because of the shape of the medial articular surfaces of the femur and tibia. The medial femoral condyle continues to slide a little, after the lateral femoral condyle has used up all its joint surface. The rotation takes place around the centre of the lateral tibial condyle. Since the lateral meniscus is circular this presents no problem. This final movement of medial rotation, just as the knee reaches full extension, has the effect of placing the knee in the position of **ligament tension**. The joint is said to be **locked** in the **close packed position**. The **anterior cruciate, posterior capsule** and **oblique ligament**, as well as the **collateral ligaments**, are all tight. The knee is therefore stable and strong and able to bear the weight of the upright body above, with minimal energy expenditure (Fig. 10.23).

When flexing the knee from the straight-legged position the joint has first to be unlocked by lateral rotation of the femur on the tibia. A small muscle called the **popliteus** is responsible for this (Fig. 10.17). This muscle arises from the posterior surface of the tibia and is covered by an expansion of the semimembranosus. It passes upwards and laterally, and enters the knee joint by passing through a hole in the joint capsule. Its insertion is into the lateral femoral condyle. It can laterally rotate the femur on the tibia. It is also said to give a few fibres to the lateral meniscus. This would account for some of the increased mobility of this meniscus (see below). Flexion of the straight leg, therefore, starts with a small lateral rotation of the femur to 'unlock' the joint. This is brought about by the popliteus and then flexion continues through the action of biceps, semitendinosus and semimembranosus. The four muscles inserted into the tibia, gracilis, sartorius, semimembranosus and semitendinosus can also produce medial rotation of the tibia. Only the biceps, which is inserted into the fibula, can produce lateral rotation of the lower leg at the knee joint. The important relationships of the knee joint are found behind: the neurovascular structures in the popliteal fossa are closely related to the capsule of the joint in this region.

Applied anatomy of the knee joint

Injuries to knee joints are common. The most frequent things injured are the **ligaments** and the **menisci**. The knee joint reacts to injury by an outpouring of synovial fluid. A swollen knee results and, since the

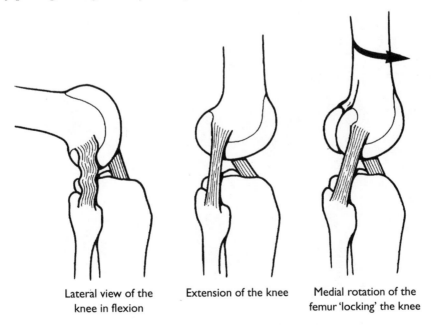

Lateral view of the knee in flexion   Extension of the knee   Medial rotation of the femur 'locking' the knee

Figure 10.23 In flexion, the fibular and tibial collateral ligaments are slack. As the knee comes into extension they tighten along with the anterior cruciate. The lateral femoral condyle then rotates on the circular lateral meniscus as the medial femoral condyle continues to move. In full extension, the knee is 'locked' and all ligaments are in tension.

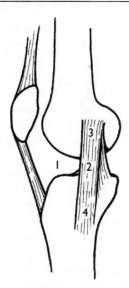

Figure 10.24 Following injury to the medial meniscus points 1 and 2 are commonly tender. When there has been ligament injury, points 3 and 4 are usually the most painful on examination.

suprapatella bursa communicates with the synovial membrane of the knee joint, there is also frequently diffuse swelling above the knee. One ligament commonly injured is the **tibial collateral ligament**. This frequently occurs during twisting sprains at the knee and is often combined with injury to the **medial meniscus**. The medial meniscus is more frequently injured, partly because it is not so mobile or so circular in shape as the lateral. Often, immediately after such an injury, the split medial meniscus prevents full extension of the knee. The joint is said to be locked due to the torn piece of cartilage getting caught between the articulating surfaces. If the knee is examined, the points of tenderness are often those shown in Figure 10.24. A more severe form of injury often tears the anterior cruciate ligament. The resulting injury is often called the 'unhappy triad' – tibial collateral ligament, medial meniscus and anterior cruciate ligament.

chapter 11

The Leg, Ankle and Foot

The distal ends of the **tibia** and **fibula** articulate with the bones of the **ankle**. The shaft of the tibia presents a very sharp anterior border (Fig. 11.1). This lies subcutaneously and can easily be palpated. Laterally, facing the fibula, there is another sharp edge called the **interosseous border**. A transverse section of the tibia is more or less triangular in shape. The lower end of the tibia should be studied together with the lower end of the fibula for they both form an important unit at the lower end of the leg. The fibula consists of a **head** at its upper end. This articulates with the lateral tibial condyle by means of a synovial joint called the **proximal tibiofibular joint**. Below the head of the fibula is a narrower **neck**. The thin shaft of the fibula presents an interosseous border which faces the interosseous border of the tibia. The two bones are united between these borders by an **interosseous membrane**. Like the membrane found in the forearm, this also gives additional area for muscle origin. The fibres slope obliquely down from the tibia to the fibula. There is a hole in the membrane near its upper limit which transmits the **anterior tibial artery** from the popliteal fossa to the front of the leg.

The only notable landmark to be found on the posterior aspect of the tibia is the **soleal line**, an oblique impression on the back of the bone near its upper end (Fig. 11.1). Far more important are the details of the lower ends of the two bones. These are united by a strong **fibrous joint** called the **distal tibiofibular joint**. The bones are further held together by **anterior** and **posterior tibiofibular ligaments**. The posterior ligament is particularly strong and projects low down over the back of the ankle joint (Fig. 11.1). The lower surface of the tibia presents a quadrilateral articular

area and medially it projects downwards at the side of the ankle joint as the **medial malleolus**. On the lateral side, the fibula projects downwards as the **lateral malleolus**. It is at a lower level than the medial malleolus and slightly posterior to it. The malleoli and their positions can easily be palpated. It can now be seen that the malleoli, the inferior surface of the tibia and the posterior tibiofibular ligament form a **mortise** into which the upper ankle bone can fit (Fig. 11.2). The distal tibiofibular joint must be extremely strong to maintain the integrity of the mortise, otherwise the ankle bone would be forced up between the tibia and fibula during walking and running (Fig. 11.2).

The **tarsal bones** are more irregularly arranged than the more mobile carpal bones of the wrist. This irregularity is partly the result of upright bipedal locomotion which relies on a more stable arrangement of the bones. Look at the normal arrangement of these tarsal bones (Figs 11.3 and 11.4). Learn carefully the names and positions of the tarsal bones using Figures 11.3 and 11.4 and an articulated skeleton of the foot if you can. The **talus** sits at the summit. It is mounted on top of the upper surface of the heel bone or **calcaneus**. The talar articular surface fits into the ankle mortise, so forming the **ankle joint**. The articulation between the talus and the calcaneus is called the **subtalar joint**. Along the lateral edge of the foot the calcaneus articulates with the **cuboid** through the **calcaneocuboid joint**. The medial edge of the foot is raised off the ground and this section is made up of four bones. The **navicular** articulates with the talus through the **talonavicular joint** and this in turn articulates with three **cuneiforms** (medial, intermediate and lateral). Do not proceed until you feel familiar

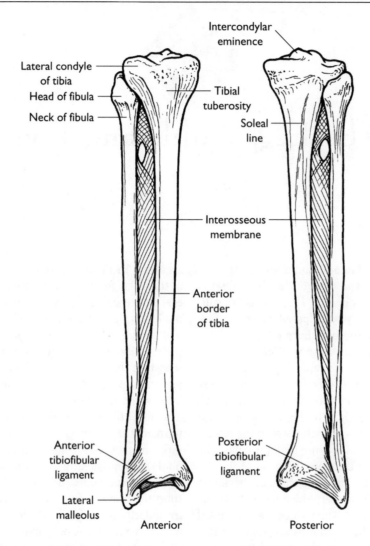

Figure 11.1   Anterior and posterior views of important bony landmarks on the tibia and fibula.

with the names and positions of the tarsal bones and the joints between them. Turn your attention to a radiograph of these bones and identify once again the tarsal bones and joints (Fig. 11.5).

In spite of the irregularity of these bones, there is a basic pattern that may be traced back to the primitive arrangement in other animals. This is interesting and offers some explanation for a seemingly complex pattern in humans. The primitive mammalian arrangement of bones in fore and hind limbs is shown in Figure 11.6. Here there are three bones in the proximal row and five in the distal row. In the centre is a central bone (C). Of the three bones in the proximal row, one lies distal to each limb bone, that is, U lies distal to the ulna or, for example, F lies distal to the fibula

and in the same way the other lies distal to the second limb bone (R is distal to the radius and T is distal to the tibia). Between the two is an intermediate bone (I). The five distal bones each articulate with a metacarpal or metatarsal. The transition from this primitive pattern to that in the human carpus and tarsus is shown in Figure 11.6. In both carpus and tarsus the 4th and 5th bones of the distal row have fused. These now form the hamate and cuboid respectively. These bones therefore articulate with two metacarpals or metatarsals. Bones C and R unite to form the scaphoid in the wrist. In the tarsus, T forms the talus and F the calcaneus. Bone I is represented simply by a small tubercle of the talus, and bone C becomes the navicular.

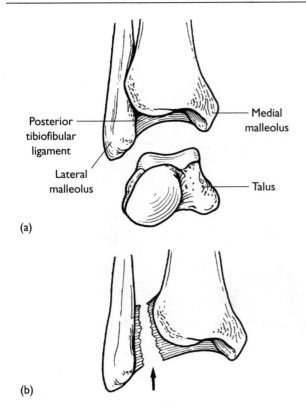

(a)

Posterior tibiofibular ligament

Lateral malleolus

Medial malleolus

Talus

(b)

Figure 11.2 (a) The malleoli, inferior surface of the tibia and the posterior tibiofibular ligament form a mortise into which the talus fits. (b) Extreme force, displacing the talus upwards, results in rupture of the distal tibiofibular joint.

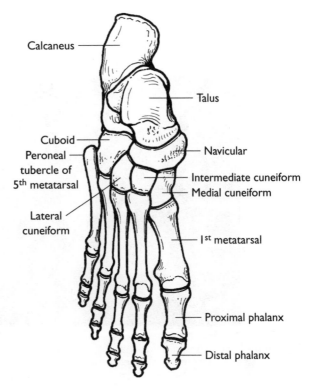

Calcaneus

Talus

Cuboid

Peroneal tubercle of 5th metatarsal

Lateral cuneiform

Navicular

Intermediate cuneiform

Medial cuneiform

1st metatarsal

Proximal phalanx

Distal phalanx

Figure 11.3 The bones of the foot seen from above.

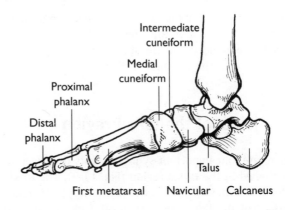

Intermediate cuneiform

Medial cuneiform

Proximal phalanx

Distal phalanx

Talus

First metatarsal   Navicular   Calcaneus

Figure 11.4 The bones of the foot seen from the medial side.

The arrangement of the tarsal bones ensures that the body weight is transmitted in an even and acceptable manner. The **talus** is the first to transmit the weight through itself to two bony pillars which rest on the ground. It is therefore from this point of view a little like the **keystone** of a Roman arch (Fig. 11.7). The posterior pillar or **ray** is composed of the calcaneus and the anterior pillar or ray is made up of the navicular and the three cuneiforms. The arch so formed is called the **longitudinal arch of the foot**. The arch is maintained by the shape of the bones, by the action of small muscles and by strong ligaments and tendons. During running, the longitudinal arch is compressed by about 1 cm towards the ground. This stretches the **long** and **short plantar ligaments** that span the arch beneath. These ligaments store energy like stretched elastic and then recoil as the foot leaves the ground, returning over 70% of their stored energy.

The bony framework of the lateral side of the foot is composed of the **cuboid**, and 4th and 5th metatar-

sals. This **lateral ray** does not in fact take much weight when standing; it is more a balancing part of the foot but it bears weight momentarily during walking. It lies in gentle contact with the ground when standing, there being no longitudinal arch on this side of the foot. (Fig. 11.8).

Place your foot on the ground as when walking. Notice that at **heel strike** the weight of the body passes through the heel. Next, body weight is spread over the lateral aspect of the foot forwards, to the

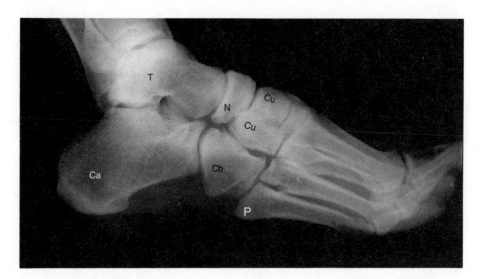

Figure 11.5   The bones of the foot as they appear on a radiograph. T, talus; N, navicular; Cu, cuneiforms; Ca, calcaneus; Cb, cuboid; P, peroneal tubercle of 5th metatarsal.

heads of the metatarsals. Then it is rolled across these to the 'ball of the foot' and the head of the 1st metatarsal. **Toe off** occurs as the stout powerful big toe or **hallux** propels the body forwards (Fig. 11.8).

The joints of the tarsal region

There are four important synovial joints that need to be studied in the tarsal region (Fig. 11.9). The **ankle joint** is a synovial joint between the upper articular surface of the talus and the mortise formed by the tibia and fibula. The upper articular surface of the talus is called the **trochlea**. From the side it looks very much like a section of a cylinder (Fig. 11.10). This articulating surface fits into the mortise formed by the lower surface of the tibia and the medial and lateral malleoli (Fig. 11.11). The upper surface of the trochlea articulates with the lower tibial surface and the articular surfaces of the malleoli with the sides of the trochlea. In some tali, the trochlea narrows towards the back. The ankle is a **hinge joint**. When the foot is at right angles to the leg, the ankle joint is said to be in the neutral position (Fig. 11.12). When the foot

moves so that the toes point down the joint is said to be **plantar flexed** (Fig. 11.12). Movement of the foot upwards is called **dorsiflexion**. The malleoli hold the sides of the talus, pinching it and holding it steady during the movements of plantar and dorsiflexion. If the talus is of the type that narrows it might be imagined that in plantarflexion, when the narrow posterior part of the trochlea is between the malleoli, there would be some 'looseness' in the joint. This is not the case. The inferior tibiofibular ligament is able to stretch a little and the fibula to bend. The mortise holds the talus firm in plantarflexion and then, as the wider parts of the trochlea pass through the mortise, the malleoli separate a millimetre or two to accommodate it.

The fibrous capsule of the ankle joint is strong and attached to the articular margins. At the back this is strengthened as the posterior tibiofibular ligament. On either side it is also strengthened by ligaments (see below). The synovial membrane lines all non-articular surfaces in the joint.

The **subtalar joint** is an important synovial joint. The articular surface of the calcaneus is dome shaped and curved. This combination ensures that the calcaneus moves under the talus in a particular way

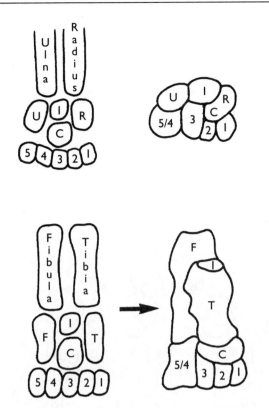

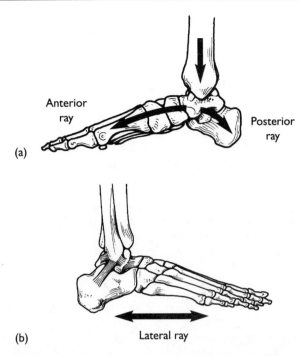

Figure 11.7 (a) The talus transmits the weight of the foot through the anterior and posterior rays of the longitudinal arch of the foot. (b) The lateral ray bears weight through the cuboid and the 4th and 5th metatarsals, on the lateral side of the foot.

Figure 11.6 It is possible to trace the regular arrangement of the bones of the carpus and tarsus in primitive mammals through to the seemingly irregular arrangement in modern humans.

(Figs 11.13 and 11.14). Point the big toe of your left foot away from the midline of the body as in (A) of Figure 11.14. This movement is called **abduction**. Notice that at the same time the lateral edge of the foot is raised, a movement called **eversion**. Movement in the opposite direction as in (C) in Figure 11.14 is **adduction**, and is accompanied by a raising of the medial edge of the foot called **inversion**. Much of these combination movements of **inversion/adduction** and **eversion/abduction** come about because of the peculiar shape of the articular surfaces of the subtalar joint. This shape is best seen on the upper surface of the calcaneus after removal of the talus (Fig. 11.15).

The **talonavicular joint** is a ball and socket type of synovial joint (Fig. 11.9). The ball is the **head of the talus** and the socket is formed from the **sustentaculum tali** and the **navicular**. Between these two bones is a ligament called the **spring ligament** (Figs 11.15 and 11.16). The sustentaculum is a bony platform on the medial side of the calcaneus. Although the talonavicular joint is a ball and socket type, it certainly does not exhibit the typical free movements of this sort of

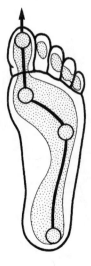

Figure 11.8 Weight is borne by the calcaneus at heel strike. It then rolls over the lateral aspect of the foot, across the heads of the metatarsals to the ball of the foot on the medial side and subsequently through the big toe at toe off.

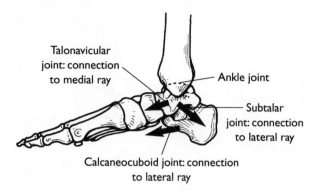

Talonavicular joint: connection to medial ray

Ankle joint

Subtalar joint: connection to lateral ray

Calcaneocuboid joint: connection to lateral ray

Figure 11.9   The ankle joint, the subtalar joint, the calcaneocuboid joint and the talonavicular joint are the four important synovial joints in the ankle region.

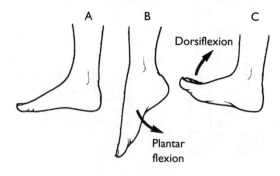

Dorsiflexion

Plantar flexion

Figure 11.12   The ankle is a hinge joint and in (A) it is in the neutral position. In (B) the ankle is plantarflexed and the toes point downwards; in (C) the ankle is dorsiflexed.

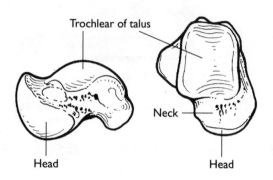

Trochlear of talus

Neck

Head

Head

Figure 11.10   The talus seen from the side and from above.

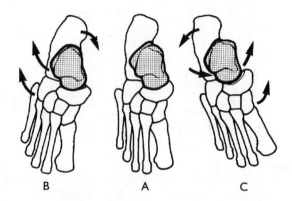

B   A   C

Figure 11.13   There is a dome-shaped joint between the calcaneus and talus. The joint between the talus and navicular form a shallow ball and socket joint. In (A), (B) and (C) the talus is stationary and the calcaneus with the rest of the foot moves beneath this and swings either into abduction/eversion (A) or adduction/inversion (C).

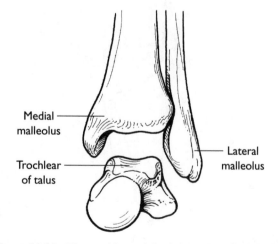

Medial malleolus

Trochlear of talus

Lateral malleolus

Figure 11.11   The trochlear of the talus articulates into the mortise formed by the lower surfaces of the tibia and fibula and the malleoli.

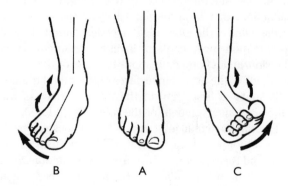

B   A   C

Figure 11.14   Seen from the front, it is clear that the lateral border of the foot rises in eversion/abduction and that the medial border of the foot rises in adduction/inversion.

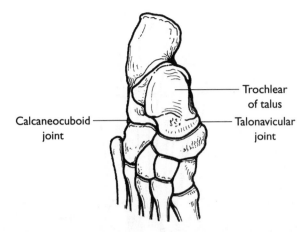

Figure 11.15 The head of the talus overlies the sustentaculum tali of the calcaneus and abuts into the navicular. It forms a ball and socket type of joint with both of these bones.

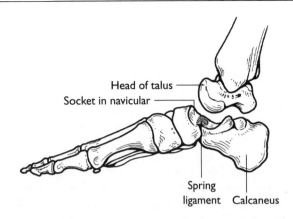

Figure 11.16 Disarticulation of the talonavicular joint reveals the spring ligament between the calcaneus and navicular.

joint. The movements at the joint are those of the tarsus swinging into **inversion/adduction** and **eversion/abduction** beneath the talus.

The **calcaneocuboid joint** is a synovial joint. The articular surfaces are rather flat and the movements that occur are those of slight gliding of one surface on the other. In summary the movements of the **subtalar** and **transverse tarsal** joints are those of **inversion/adduction** or **eversion/abduction**. They also contribute to the pliability of the tarsus.

Ligaments around the tarsal joints

The ligaments around the tarsus often strengthen one or more joints; it is thus easier to study them after the four main joints have been described. The **medial ligament** is triangular in shape (and is therefore sometimes called the **deltoid ligament**), its apex being attached to the medial malleolus (Fig. 11.17). Its base is attached to the talus and therefore it spans the **ankle joint**, supporting its medial aspect. However, the base also gains attachment to the calcaneus along

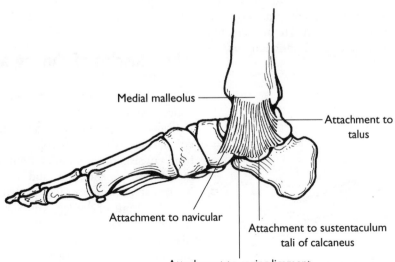

Figure 11.17 The base of the deltoid ligament, or medial ligament of the ankle, attaches to the navicular, spring ligament and sustentaculum tali of the calcaneus.

the sustentaculum tali. It therefore also spans the **subtalar joint** by means of these fibres. Similarly, the anterior fibres of the ligament attach to the spring ligament and navicular. By doing this it is also supporting the 'socket' of the **talonavicular joint.**

The **lateral ligament** of the ankle joint is also strong and often sprained with injuries of the ankle. It is formed from three radiating fibrous bands (Fig. 11.18). The anterior and posterior bands span the gap between the lateral malleolus and the anterior and posterior aspects of the lateral talar surface respectively. They thus strengthen the lateral side of the ankle joint. The middle band passes downwards and backwards to the calcaneus. It therefore spans both ankle and subtalar joints, and therefore stabilizes both of these articulations.

The **long plantar ligament** is found in the sole of the foot (Fig. 11.19). It arises from the inferior surface of the calcaneus and extends under the surface of the cuboid and then forwards to the base of the metatarsals laterally. It supports the other main joint that has been studied, the **calcaneocuboid joint**. The rest of the tarsal bones are also united by synovial joints, but these have much less clinical importance. **Tarsometatarsal, metatarsophalangeal** and **interphalangeal joints** are also all synovial. Perhaps the most interesting and important of these is the metatarsophalangeal joint of the big toe. The reason is, quite apart from its role in walking, that it is frequently the site of arthritis and occasionally gout. Notice that, in comparison with the MCP and IP joints of the hand, the corresponding joints of the foot can only perform the movements of flexion and extension. The movements of abduction, adduction and circumduction *can* be

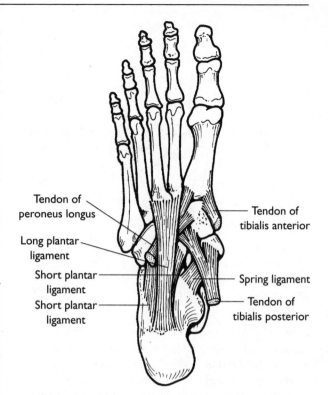

Figure 11.19   The long and short plantar ligaments run forwards from the calcaneus. The tendon of peroneus longus grooves the cuboid as it runs between these two plantar ligaments. The spring ligament is also seen from below here.

produced in the metatarsophalangeal joints but only passively.

The muscles of the leg and foot

Below the knee joint, the musculature of the leg is concerned with movements of the ankle and toes. Consider this part of the leg as being divided into two compartments by an osseofascial 'septum'. The 'septum' consists of the **tibia** and **fibula** connected by an **interosseous membrane** and a so-called **posterior intermuscular septum** (Fig. 11.20).

At the front of the leg, anterior to the osseofascial septum, lies a mass of muscle which functions to **dorsiflex** the ankle and **extend** the toes. As well as this function, the most medial muscle also produces **inversion/adduction** of the foot, whereas on the lateral side two muscles of the group possess the function of **eversion/abduction**. All the muscles on the

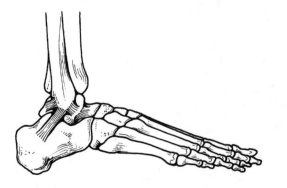

Figure 11.18   The lateral ligament of the ankle is formed from three fibrous bands. The posterior and anterior bands run from the malleolus to the lateral talar surface. The middle band runs posteroinferiorly to the calcaneus.

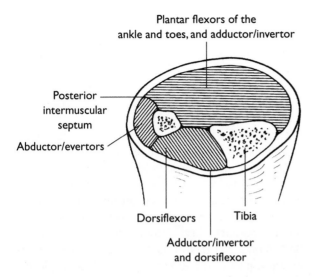

Figure 11.20 Osseofascial septa divide the leg into compartments.

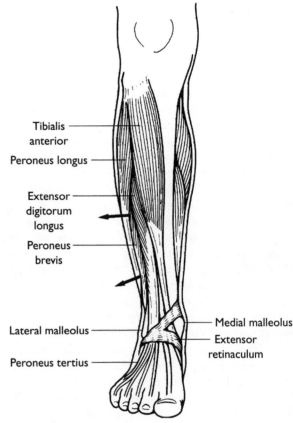

Figure 11.21 The muscles of the front of the leg and the extensor retinaculum.

front of the leg are supplied by the **common peroneal branch** of the sciatic nerve.

At the back of the leg, behind the osseofascial septum, lies a great mass of muscle concerned with **plantar flexion** at the ankle and **flexion of the toes**. The tendons of these muscles pass to the heel and into the sole of the foot. One muscle of the calf is also an **adductor/invertor**. The musculature at the back of the leg is supplied by the **tibial branch** of the sciatic nerve.

The muscles of the front of the leg

The centrally positioned muscles of this group are responsible for extension of the toes. Since they also pass across the ankle joint, they also have a subsidiary function of dorsiflexion at the ankle. The muscles are the **extensor digitorum longus** and the **extensor hallucis longus**. As they pass over the front of the ankle they are held down by thickenings in the deep fascia called the **extensor retinacula** (Fig. 11.21). The superior of these retinacula extends between the tibia and fibula. The inferior retinaculum is usually 'Y' shaped. The stem of the 'Y' is attached to the lateral side of the calcaneus. The upper limb attaches to the medial malleolus and the lower limb sweeps around the medial border of the foot to blend with the deep fascia in the sole (Fig. 11.21).

The **extensor digitorum longus** arises from the fibula. As it approaches the ankle it gives a tendon that passes deep to the extensor retinacula. As it passes deep to these structures it is covered with a synovial sheath. The tendon divides into four slips which pass towards the four lateral toes. Over the proximal phalanges these tendons form **extensor expansions** similar to those found in the fingers. A central slip, thereafter, gains insertion into the base of the middle phalanx and two collateral slips extend into the base of the distal phalanx. The action of the extensor digitorum longus is to extend the interphalangeal and metatarsophalangeal joints of the lateral four toes. The nerve supply of the muscle comes from the **deep peroneal nerve**.

The **extensor hallucis longus** arises from the mid-fibular shaft and interosseous membrane. While passing deep to the extensor retinacula its tendon is surrounded by a synovial sheath. Its long, strong tendon is inserted into the base of the distal phalanx of the big toe. Its action therefore is to extend the interphalangeal and metatarsophalangeal joints of this toe. It is supplied by the **deep peroneal nerve**. Occasionally, this tendon may be ruptured during injury. It will then be impossible to extend the big toe, which lies in a flexed position. Walking without shoes is then difficult since the flexed toe tends to trip the patient up. These two muscles, the extensor digitorum longus and extensor hallucis longus, are assisted by a small muscle found on the dorsum of the foot. This muscle is the **extensor digitorum brevis/hallucis brevis** (Fig. 11.22). It arises from the upper surface of the calcaneus and divides into four tendons. The most medial of these is the **extensor hallucis brevis**. It passes to the proximal phalanx of the big toe. The other three gain insertion into the extensor expansions of the 2nd, 3rd and 4th toes. This muscle also is supplied by the **deep peroneal nerve**.

In the foot, as in the hand, there are **lumbrical** and **interosseous** muscles. However, their function is far less important. The lumbricals arise from the long flexor tendons in the sole of the foot and the interossei from the metatarsal bones. Their delicate tendons insert into the extensor expansions of the 2nd, 3rd, 4th and 5th toes. Their action in the foot is to flex the metatarsophalangeal joints and weakly to extend the interphalangeal joints. Details of these muscle origins in the sole of the foot are not important.

The most medial muscle in the front of the leg is large. It arises from the tibia and interosseous membrane and is called the **tibialis anterior** (Fig. 11.21). The tendon passes deep to the extensor retinacula where it is of course covered with a synovial sheath.

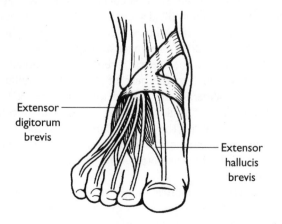

Figure 11.22 The extensor digitorum brevis/hallucis brevis splits into four tendons, the most medial of which runs to the great toe.

Extensor digitorum brevis

Extensor hallucis brevis

It is inserted into the medial side of the foot into the medial cuneiform and first metatarsal. As well as dorsiflexing the foot at the ankle joint, the muscle is also an **invertor/adductor** of the foot, that is, it lifts the medial border of the foot and points the big toe towards the midline of the body. If you perform this movement with your own foot you will see the tibialis anterior tendon standing out. The muscle once again is supplied by the **deep peroneal nerve**.

The most lateral muscles in front of the leg are the **peroneal muscles** (Fig. 11.21). The peroneal muscles perform the functions of **eversion/abduction**. The **peroneus longus** arises from the upper part of the fibula and the **peroneus brevis** from lower down the fibula. Both tendons curl around the lateral malleolus and lateral aspect of the ankle. They are held in place in this region by two retinacula, the **superior** and **inferior peroneal retinacula** (Fig. 11.23). The superior retinaculum bridges the gap between the lateral malleolus and calcaneus. The inferior is attached at both its ends to the lateral surface of the calcaneus. The two peroneal tendons pass deep to both of these retinacula. Deep to the superior they are covered by a common synovial sheath, but deep to the inferior retinaculum the tendons are covered with separate sheaths. The brevis is inserted into the peroneal tubercle at the base of the 5th metatarsal. The longus sweeps around into the sole of the foot. Here it passes towards the medial border and inserts into the same bones as the tibialis anterior, medial cuneiform and 1st metatarsal (Fig. 11.24). These two tendons (tibialis anterior and peroneus longus), pulling opposite ways on the same insertions, are the great **evertor/abductor** and **invertor/adductor** muscles of the foot. As the peroneus longus passes through the sole of the foot it is held in a groove in the cuboid by the long plantar ligament (Fig. 11.19). Here it is surrounded by a synovial sheath. Both **peroneal muscles** are supplied by the **superficial peroneal nerve**. Occasionally there is a small muscular slip called the **peroneus tertius**. This inconstant muscle is really a slip of extensor digitorum longus and arises from the lower fibula, but its delicate tendon does not pass through the peroneal retinacula. It passes deep to the extensor retinaculum. Like the peroneus brevis it goes to the base of the 5th metatarsal. It is supplied, along with the other muscles of the extensor retinacula, by the deep peroneal nerve and functions with these as a weak dorsiflexor.

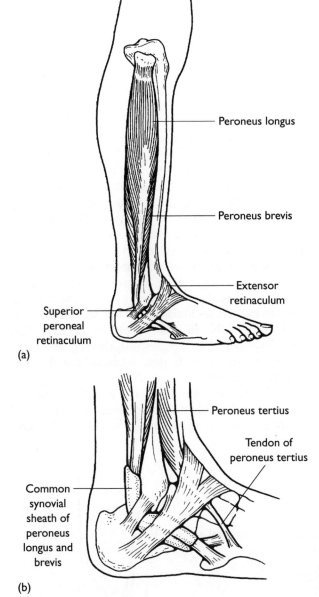

(a)

(b)

Figure 11.23 The peroneus longus and brevis arise from the fibula (a) and run beneath the superior and inferior peroneal retinacula (b). They evert/abduct the foot.

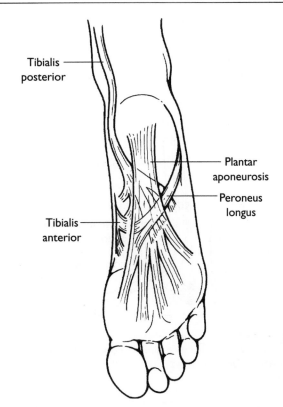

Figure 11.24 The peroneus longus sweeps under the foot towards the tibialis anterior. These two muscles then pull in opposite ways.

The neurovascular supply to the front of the leg

The nerve supplying the muscles at the front of the leg is the **common peroneal branch** of the sciatic nerve. The arterial supply comes from the **anterior tibial branch** of the **popliteal artery**. The **common** **peroneal nerve** was last identified as it was leaving the popliteal fossa. Here, at the lateral side of the knee, it comes to lie on the neck of the fibula. It can be rolled on the bone at this site. It divides into **deep** and **superficial peroneal branches**. These are mixed nerves supplying between them all the muscles and skin on the front of the leg. The deep peroneal nerve passes on to the front of the interosseous membrane. It may be found in this position by separating the tibialis anterior from the extensor digitorum and extensor hallucis longus (Fig 11.25 and 11.26). Near the ankle it is crossed by the tendon of the extensor hallucis longus as that tendon passes to the big toe. On the dorsum of the foot, therefore, it lies between the tendons of extensor digitorum longus and extensor hallucis longus. Here it ends by dividing into lateral and medial branches. The lateral division supplies the extensor digitorum brevis and the medial division is cutaneous, supplying the 1st cleft skin. While in the front of the leg the deep peroneal nerve supplies the extensor digitorum longus and brevis, and the extensor hallucis longus and tibialis anterior.

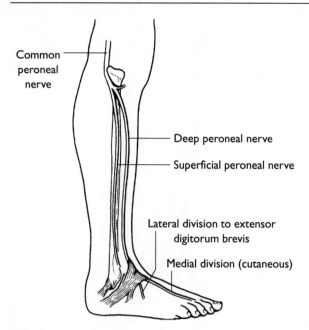

Figure 11.25   The common peroneal nerve runs beneath the head of the fibula and then divides into the deep peroneal and superficial peroneal nerves.

The superficial peroneal nerve immediately passes into the substance of the peroneus longus and then into the peroneus brevis. It supplies only these two muscles. What is left of the nerve are sensory neurons that emerge in the lower leg as a nerve that divides into lateral and medial branches. These supply skin on the dorsum of the foot and toes as shown in Figure 11.27.

The **anterior tibial artery** is a branch of the popliteal artery. It enters the front of the leg by piercing the interosseous membrane (Fig. 11.1). Here it joins the deep peroneal nerve and passes with it down the leg. It supplies the muscles of the front of the leg with blood. It passes deep to the extensor retinacula with the deep peroneal nerve and can be easily felt in the limb about midway between the malleoli, that is, between the extensor hallucis longus and the extensor digitorum longus. The hallucis tendon is easily identifed if the subject is asked to extend the big toe. This artery becomes important to the diagnostician in assessment of the vascular supply to the foot. The artery is renamed as it passes into this region on the dorsum of the foot. It now becomes the **dorsalis pedis** (Fig. 11.28).

On the dorsum of the foot the vessel runs to the first web space with the medial branch of the deep peroneal nerve. It then enters the sole of the foot

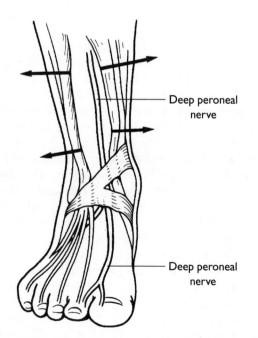

Figure 11.26   The deep peroneal nerve lies between (and supplies) tibialis anterior medially and extensor digitorum and extensor hallucis longus laterally. It runs beneath the extensor retinaculum and continues on to supply the skin of the first cleft.

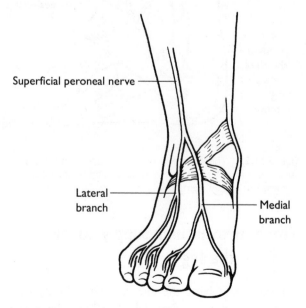

Figure 11.27   The superficial peroneal nerve runs superficial to the extensor retinaculum. Its medial and lateral branches supply the skin on the dorsum of the foot and toes.

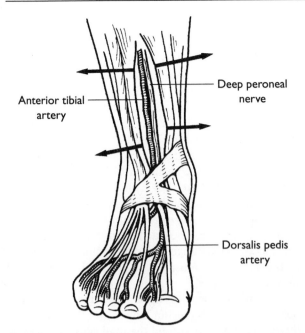

Figure 11.28 The anterior tibial artery runs with the deep peroneal nerve. It becomes the dorsalis pedis artery on the dorsum of the foot where it can be felt as a foot pulse.

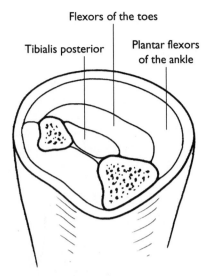

Figure 11.29 The muscles of the flexor compartment of the leg are arranged in three layers.

where it supplies some of its blood. On the dorsum it gives an arcuate branch which supplies metatarsals and toes by means of dorsal metatarsal and digital branches.

The muscles at the back of the leg

The muscles of the calf are concerned with **plantar flexion** of the foot at the ankle and **flexion** of the toes. The muscles of this flexor compartment are arranged in three layers like 'onion skins'. Lying in the deepest stratum, and arising from the tibia and fibula and interosseous membrane, is the large **tibialis posterior**. In the middle stratum lie the **long flexors of the toes**. In the superficial layer lie the **flexor muscles of the ankle** (Fig. 11.29). The insertions of the three groups are obviously different. The tibialis posterior inserts into the sole of the foot, the toe flexors into the toes, and the superficial plantar flexors into the heel. The tendons of the first two groups reach the sole and toes by curling around the medial malleolus. A thickening of the deep fascia in this region holds the tendons in place. It is called the **flexor retinaculum** and stretches between the medial malleolus and the calcaneus

(Fig. 11.30). All the muscles of the back of the leg are supplied by branches of the **tibial nerve**.

We need to study the muscles of the three strata in a little more detail. The deepest stratum of musculature at the back of the leg consists of the **tibialis**

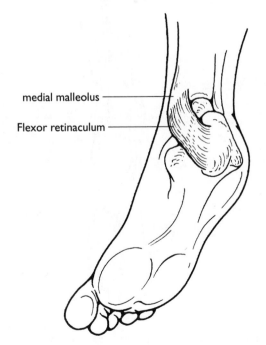

Figure 11.30 The flexor retinaculum runs between the medial malleolus and the calcaneus.

posterior (Fig. 11.31). The muscle arises from the tibia, fibula and interosseous membrane. Its tendon passes deep to the flexor retinaculum and here it is surrounded by a synovial sheath. In the sole of the foot it sends fibrous insertions to almost all of the bones in the sole; however, its chief insertion is into the navicular. Its action is to **plantar flex** the foot at the ankle but, by its pull on the medially placed navicular, it also helps to **invert/adduct** the foot. It is supplied by the **tibial nerve**.

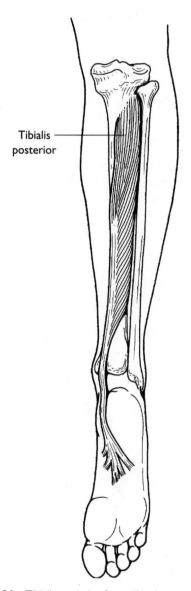

Tibialis posterior

Figure 11.31 Tibialis posterior forms the deepest layer of the muscles in the calf. It runs deep to the flexor retinaculum and into the sole of the foot.

The middle layer of musculature includes the long flexor of the toes and the long flexor of the big toe. These muscles are called the **flexor digitorum longus** and **flexor hallucis longus** respectively. Since they are the 'second skin' over the deep muscles they must arise further out from the tibia and fibula. The flexor digitorum longus arises from the tibia and the hallucis longus from the fibula. They both pass deep to the flexor retinaculum and are covered here with synovial sheaths (Fig. 11.32). The flexor digitorum longus tendon divides into four slips which insert into the terminal phalanges of the lateral four toes. The tendon of the hallucis longus inserts into the terminal phalanx of the big toe. Their actions are therefore to flex the metatarsophalangeal and interphalangeal joints of the toes. Both muscles are supplied by the **tibial nerve**.

It is useful to localize the three tendons of Tibialis posterior, flexor Digitorum longus and flexor Hallucis longus as they curl around the malleolus by referring to them as Tom, Dick and Harry! In this way you will always remember the order of tendons as they lie deep to the flexor retinaculum (Fig. 11.32).

From the medial side of each tendon of the flexor digitorum longus a **lumbrical muscle** arises. As in the palm, these muscles wind around the side of their respective metatarsophalangeal joint to insert into the extensor expansion. They assist in flexion of the metatarsophalangeal joints. However, their importance in the foot is obviously much less than in the hand. As the tendons to the toes pass along the plantar surfaces of the toes they are held in place by **fibrous flexor sheaths**. A similar arrangement was seen with the passage of the flexor tendons in the fingers. Obviously, they are also surrounded by synovial sheaths during their passage through the toe sheaths.

One further point needs to be noticed with respect to the passage of the flexor digitorum longus tendons in the sole. The tendon will obviously exert a very oblique pull as it passes from medial malleolus through the sole. In order to 'centre' the tendons in the sole a small muscle called the **flexor accessorius** arises from the calcaneus and inserts into the tendon of flexor digitorum longus.

The superficial muscles at the back of the leg are concerned with **plantar flexion of the foot at the ankle**. They are the **soleus**, the **gastrocnemius** and the **plantaris**. They are all inserted as a common tendon into the calcaneus.

The soleus is the deepest of the muscles and arises

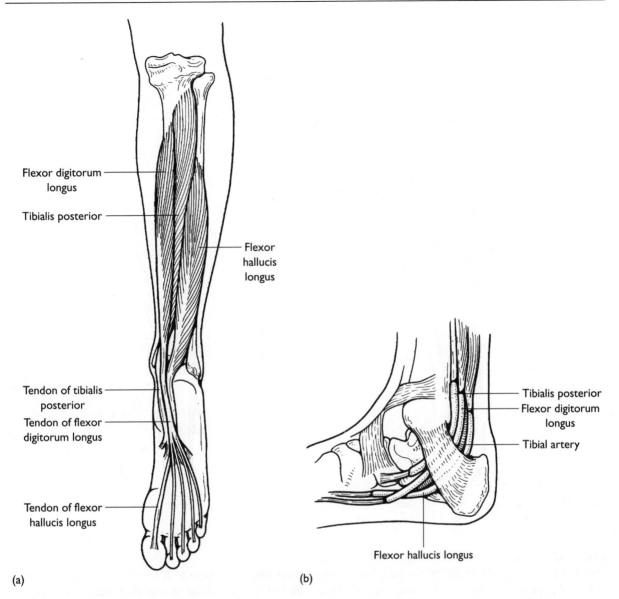

Flexor digitorum longus

Tibialis posterior

Flexor hallucis longus

Tendon of tibialis posterior

Tendon of flexor digitorum longus

Tendon of flexor hallucis longus

(a)

Tibialis posterior

Flexor digitorum longus

Tibial artery

Flexor hallucis longus

(b)

Figure 11.32 Flexor hallucis longus and flexor digitorum longus arise, respectively, lateral to and medial to tibialis posterior in the calf (a). In (b) these tendons can be seen contained within synovial sheaths running deep to the flexor retinaculum.

from the tibia and fibula. On the tibia it arises from the **soleal line** as well as from the back of the fibula. Between these two origins it forms a fibrous arch (Fig. 11.33). Near the ankle the muscle ends in a tendon which forms part of the common insertion of the tendo calcaneus.

The gastrocnemius arises by means of two heads, one from the lateral and one from the medial femoral condyles. The muscle accounts for much of the muscle mass of the calf. On the inner side of the lateral head a small muscle arises from the femur which soon

gives way to a long, delicate tendon. This is the **plantaris** (Fig. 11.34). While the long plantaris tendon has little muscle tissue associated with it, it is stretched during walking and running exactly like a length of elastic. The plantaris tendon is able to return over 90% of the energy stored in this way during walking and running. In some animals this is a vitally important mechanism in their form of locomotion (camels and kangaroos are good examples). Gastrocnemius and plantaris merge with the soleal tendon near the ankle and the three tendons make up the

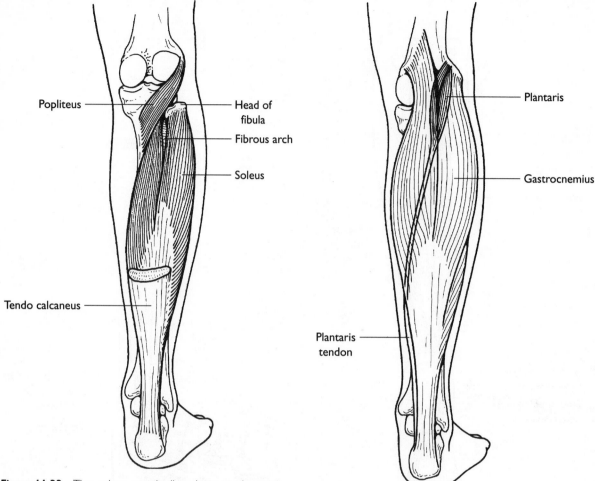

Figure 11.33 The soleus muscle lies deep to the gastrocnemius in the calf.

Figure 11.34 Plantaris is a small muscle with an extremely long tendon that runs to the tendo calcaneus.

tendo calcaneus. This tendon is inserted into the calcaneus. It can easily be felt in the limb behind the ankle. A small bursa separates the tendon from underlying bone.

All three muscles are powerful **plantar flexors** of the ankle and all are supplied by the **tibial nerve**. Study in a little more detail the tendons and muscles in the sole of the foot. These need not be learned in the same detail as the muscles in the palm of the hand. Clinically they are of much less significance.

The deepest layer of tendon and ligament in the sole has already been partially studied (Fig. 11.19). It consists of the tendons of **tibialis posterior** and **peroneus longus**. The tibialis posterior inserts into the navicular and then sends insertions into many of the other bones of the sole of the foot. The peroneus longus passes obliquely across the sole deep to the

long plantar ligament. It inserts into the medial border of the foot, that is, into the base of the big toe metatarsal and the medial cuneiform. (This is the same insertion as the tibialis anterior.) To this layer we must add some muscles that are found between the metatarsal bones. These are the **interossei**. Like those of the hand, the muscles in the foot also arise as two groups. Both groups insert into the extensor expansions of the toes. Their details need not be learned since in humans their only function is flexion of the metatarsophalangeal joints. They perform infinitely less precisely than those of the hand and fingers. The deepest layer of the sole consists therefore of the tendons of **tibialis posterior**, the **peroneus longus** and the **long plantar ligament**. The layer is completed by the metatarsals with their **interossei** (Fig. 11.35).

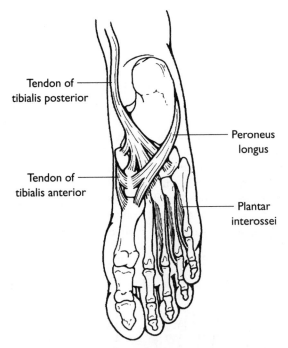

Figure 11.35 The deepest layer of the sole consists of the tendons of peroneus longus, tibialis anterior and posterior, and the plantar interossei.

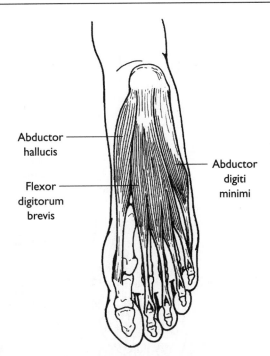

Figure 11.36 The most superficial layer of muscles in the sole of the foot are the abductors of the great and little toe and flexor digitorum brevis.

The other group of tendons and muscle already studied are those of the flexors of the toes, the **flexor digitorum longus** with its **accessorius** and the **flexor hallucis longus** (Fig. 11.37). This layer is of course superficial to the previous layer described. There are other **small muscles** found in the sole of the foot. They form **two further layers**, one being the most superficial and the other lying between the two groups described above (consult Figures 11.35 to 11.38). The details of these small muscles are given only for the sake of completeness in this text and their details need not be learned.

The most superficial group of muscles arises from the calcaneus, the short abductors inserting into the proximal phalanges of the big and 5th toes (Fig. 11.36). Between them, the flexor digitorum **brevis**, like the **superficialis** in the hand, divides into four tendons which enter the fibrous flexor sheaths of the lateral four toes. Here they split to allow the tendons of the flexor digitorum longus to pass onwards to the distal phalanges. The tendons of the brevis insert into the middle phalanges (Fig. 11.36).

The next layer is formed by the tendons of the flexor digitorum longus and flexor hallucis longus (Fig. 11.37). The third layer consists of the short

flexors of the big and 5th toes which insert into the proximal phalanges of the great and 5th toes respectively (Fig. 11.38). The **adductor hallucis**, like the adductor pollicis of the hand, arises from metatarsals and inserts into the proximal phalanx of the big toe (Fig. 11.38).

The deepest layer consists of the metatarsals and interossei (Fig. 11.35). The essential thing to grasp is the similarity in plan between the palm of the hand and the sole of the foot.

The skin and subcutaneous fat of the sole of the foot is thick, especially in the weight-bearing areas. The deep fascia is thickened into a **plantar aponeurosis**. This covers the intermediate compartment of the sole just as the palmar aponeurosis of the palm does.

Neurovascular structures of the leg and sole of the foot

We last saw the sciatic nerve in the popliteal fossa. It divides here, or even above this level, into two terminal branches, the common peroneal and the tibial nerves. It is the **tibial nerve** that is responsible for the

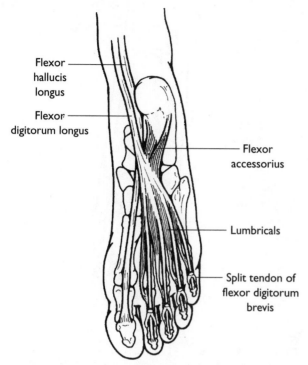

Flexor hallucis longus

Flexor digitorum longus

Flexor accessorius

Lumbricals

Split tendon of flexor digitorum brevis

Figure 11.37 If the most superficial layer of muscles is removed, the tendons of the flexor hallucis longus and flexor digitorum longus are revealed, together with the lumbricals and flexor accessorius.

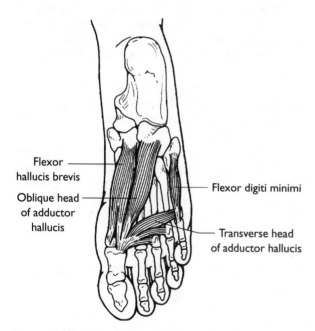

Flexor hallucis brevis

Oblique head of adductor hallucis

Flexor digiti minimi

Transverse head of adductor hallucis

Figure 11.38 Deeper still, a third layer of muscles consists of the short flexors of the toes and the two heads of adductor hallucis. Beneath this layer are the tendons and ligaments shown in Figure 11.35.

nerve supply of the muscles at the back of the leg and sole of the foot. The nerve leaves the popliteal fossa at its lower angle and immediately passes deep to the fibrous arch formed by the origin of the soleus. It therefore comes to lie deep to the most superficial stratum of muscles at the back of the leg. In this position it passes downwards in the groove between the two muscles of the middle stratum, the flexor digitorum longus and the flexor hallucis longus (Fig. 11.39). At the ankle it curls around the medial malleolus deep to the flexor retinaculum with these tendons. While under the retinaculum it divides into two terminal branches called the **medial** and **lateral plantar nerves**. Once again it is useful to compare structures in the

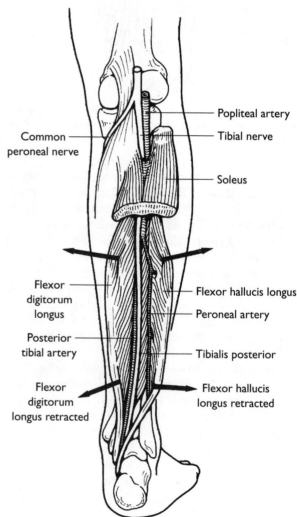

Popliteal artery

Tibial nerve

Common peroneal nerve

Soleus

Flexor digitorum longus

Flexor hallucis longus

Peroneal artery

Posterior tibial artery

Tibialis posterior

Flexor digitorum longus retracted

Flexor hallucis longus retracted

Figure 11.39 The tibial nerve runs between (and supplies) the flexor digitorum longus and flexor hallucis longus in company with the posterior tibial artery.

foot with those in the hand in order to aid the memory. The **medial plantar nerve** is the counterpart of the **median nerve** in the hand. The cutaneous supply of the two nerves is usually similar. The muscular branches are also almost similar. The median nerve supplies the **short muscles of the thumb** and the lateral **two lumbricals**. In the foot the muscular branches supply the **short muscles of the big toe** and the most **medial lumbrical**. The nerve has one other function to perform. The **flexor digitorum brevis** exists only in the sole of the foot unlike its counterpart, the flexor digitorum superficialis, which arises in the forearm. The brevis therefore needs to be supplied in the sole. The medial plantar nerve performs this function (Fig. 11.40).

The **lateral plantar nerve** is the counterpart of the **ulnar nerve**. Both divide into superficial and deep branches and the area of supply of the superficial cutaneous part is comparable (Fig. 11.41). The deep, muscular branch supplies all the other short muscles in the sole of the foot that are not supplied by the medial plantar nerve.

The blood supply of the back of the leg and sole of the foot comes from a branch of the **popliteal artery**. At the lower border of the popliteus muscle the popliteal artery divides into its two terminal branches, the **anterior and posterior tibial arteries** (Fig. 11.39). The anterior tibial artery immediately pierces the interosseous membrane and then supplies the musculature on the front of the leg. The posterior tibial artery is larger for it has a greater muscle mass to supply. It first gives a peroneal branch which passes deep to the soleal bridge to the lateral aspect of the leg. Here it supplies the peroneal muscles. The posterior tibial artery continues in company with the tibial nerve. Deep to the flexor retinaculum it divides into medial and lateral plantar arteries. These accompany the nerves of the same name. The lateral plantar artery follows the deep branch of the nerve into the depths of the sole as the so-called **plantar arch** (Fig. 11.41).

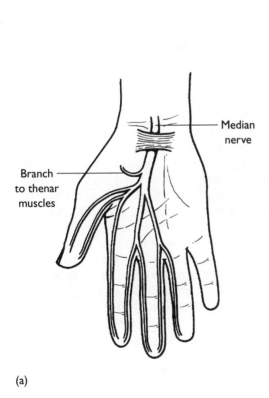

(a)

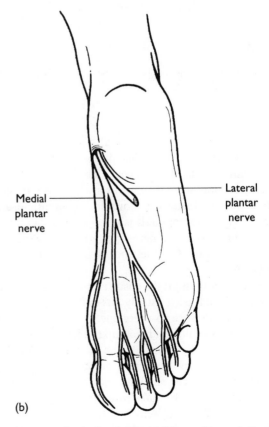

(b)

Figure 11.40 The medial plantar nerve is the counterpart of the median nerve in the hand; (a) and (b) reveal how similar this common plan really is.

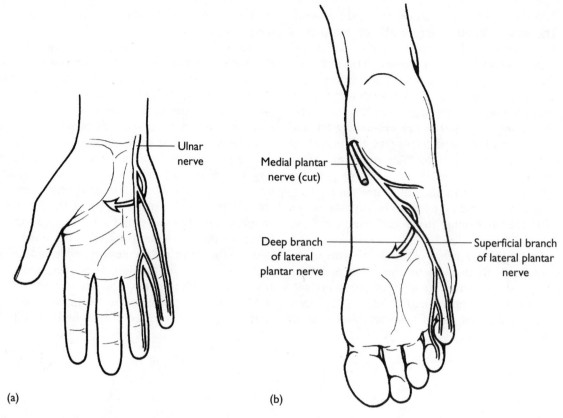

Ulnar nerve

Medial plantar nerve (cut)

Deep branch of lateral plantar nerve

Superficial branch of lateral plantar nerve

(a)   (b)

Figure 11.41   The lateral plantar nerve is the counterpart of the ulnar nerve in the hand. The similarities in their distribution are revealed in (a) and (b).

The two arteries give metatarsal and digital vessels. Their pattern need not be memorized.

Certain aspects of the lower limb are best studied when the anatomy of the limb as a whole is completed rather than by regions. Venous and lymphatic drainage are two such topics. It is also easier to obtain an overall impression of nerve patterns supplying the skin and muscles at the end of any study of the lower limb.

Because of the upright posture of humans, venous drainage from the leg usually has quite a considerable hydrostatic pressure to overcome. It often cannot be a purely passive flow of blood up the legs towards the great veins. Three things aid the flow of blood in the leg veins. Perhaps the most important is muscle movement. Muscle action massages the blood through the veins. To make sure that the blood passes in the right direction many of the leg veins contain valves. A further factor aiding the flow of venous blood is the proximity of many veins to arteries. The

pulsation of arteries also has a massaging effect. This is especially true in the case of **venae comitantes**.

In the leg blood is drained both from the superficial and deep tissues. The superficial veins lie outside the sheath of deep fascia of the leg and the deep veins course inside the sheath (Fig. 11.42). The **deep veins** are those that accompany the tibial, popliteal and femoral arteries and their branches. They take their names from the arteries that they follow. Blood flows proximally in them towards the external iliac vein. Since they are surrounded by muscles and are near pulsing arteries, blood flows efficiently in them. They are equipped with valves to maintain the correct direction of flow. The **superficial veins** have no muscular surround. They course in the subcutaneous fat. Often they do not have accompanying arteries. However, they are equipped with valves. The superficial veins drain into the deep veins by piercing the sleeve of deep fascia. At the points where they perforate they are equipped with valves to ensure that blood always

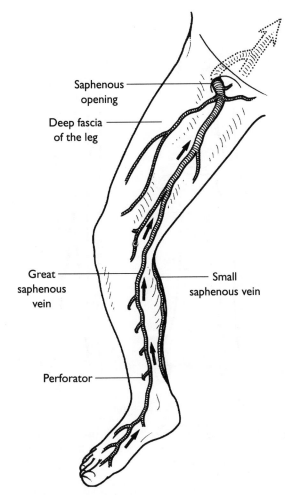

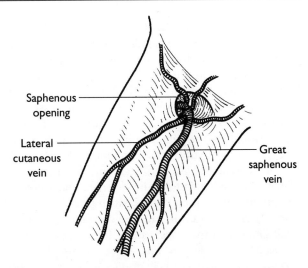

Figure 11.43 The great saphenous vein enters the saphenous opening in the cribriform fascia of the thigh.

Figure 11.42 Superficial veins in the leg lie outside the layer of deep fascia. Valves in the perforating veins ensures that flow is always from superficial veins to deeper veins.

flows from superficial to deep and not vice versa. The perforating points of these superficial veins are important because the valves in these locations prevent reflux of blood into the superficial veins. These veins are obviously not suited to venous engorgement since they are surrounded only by fat and do not accompany arteries. Excess blood in them tends to distend them and stagnate.

The two superficial veins that need to be studied in the lower limb are the **great** and **small saphenous veins**. Much of the venous blood from the sole drains through veins between the metatarsals to a subcutaneous venous arch on the dorsum of the foot. This is a similar arrangement to that seen in the palm of the hand. The reason for this is obvious. Both sole of foot and palm of hand receive pressure during grip-

ping and walking respectively. Venous drainage between the bony struts on to the dorsum is a pressure-free escape route for blood. On the medial side of the foot in the subcutaneous fat, veins converge to form the **great saphenous vein**. On the lateral side the **small saphenous vein** is formed.

The great saphenous vein drains upwards over the surface of the medial malleolus and within the subcutaneous tissues of the medial side of the leg. In the region of the ankle and lower leg there are several important perforators. It continues upwards, veering posteriorly as it negotiates the knee, and reaches the front of the thigh. During the upper part of its course it receives several tributaries. Just below the medial end of the inguinal ligament it dips into the deeper aspects of the thigh. This termination is a perforator. It enters through a hole in the deep fascia called the saphenous opening (Fig. 11.43). The condensed fascia which fills in this opening is called the **cribriform fascia**. A valve is present at this perforation as in all venous perforators.

The short saphenous vein courses from the lateral side of the ankle to the midline at the back of the lower leg. It perforates the deep fascial sleeve in the popliteal region and enters the popliteal vein.

Lymphatic drainage of the lower limb

The general rule of lymphatic pathways in the limbs is that superficial lymphatics follow veins and deep lymphatics follow arteries. Most drain along the great saphenous vein to the inguinal nodes in the groin. Not much lymph drains along the small saphenous vein. Spreading infections of the foot or lower leg are therefore followed by the appearance of tender, enlarged nodes in the inguinal group. The vessels following the great saphenous vein drain into the vertical nodes along the vein. Lymph drains into the horizontal group of superficial inguinal nodes from the lower abdominal wall and back, and from the perineum. All the lymph from the superficial nodes passes deeply through lymph vessels which pierce the cribriform fascia. They drain into the deep inguinal nodes that lie around the upper end of the femoral vein.

Deep lymphatics in the lower limb follow the arteries and also eventually drain into the deep inguinal group of nodes. All the lymph from the deep group of nodes drains into lymph vessels through the femoral canal into the abdominal cavity. Here the lymph vessels carry them along the course of the iliac arteries and eventually to the aorta, to reach the thoracic duct.

Applied anatomy of the ankle and foot

Fracture of the tibia and fibula is extremely common. Often the pattern of breakage depends on the type of force involved. For example, a car bumper striking the leg will frequently cause the bones to break at the same level (Fig. 11.44). On the other hand a twisting strain such as that incurred in many skiing accidents will cause a break at different levels (Fig. 11.44). The bones also are frequently seen broken in the region of the malleoli (Fig. 11.44). Such a fracture is called a **Pott's fracture**.

Of all the injuries that occur during sports or in everyday life, perhaps one of the commonest is the **sprained ankle**. In such an injury there is usually a forced inversion strain and the lateral ligament is either partially or completely torn. Of the three bands of the ligament, the anterior talofibular and the calcaneofibular are usually the ones injured. The posterior ligament ruptures only with the most severe type of injury involving complete disruption of the ankle.

Troubles with muscles, tendons and nerves also occur in the leg, ankle and foot. Occasionally the

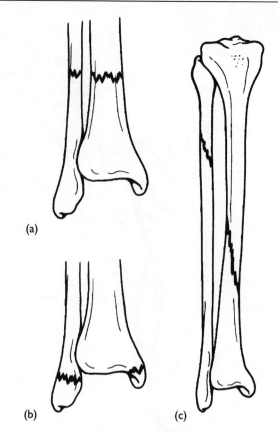

(a)

(b)   (c)

Figure 11.44   Fractures of the bones in the leg occur in one of several patterns. In (a) both are fractured at the same level. In (b) the levels are different and in (c) both malleoli are fractured (refer to text for details).

plantaris tendon ruptures spontaneously. This causes sudden severe pain in the calf. The **tendo calcaneus** can also be the site of partial or complete rupture. Poliomyelitis often affects the dorsiflexors and evertors of the leg. This is seen less nowadays following the polio vaccination programme. If a patient is badly placed on an operating table, pressure on the common peroneal nerve may result in paralysis of the muscles supplied by the nerve and the patient notices this on recovering from the anaesthetic. The trouble spot is the place where the nerve lies superficially on the neck of the fibula. A tight plaster of Paris or tourniquet in this position may have a similar effect. Any permanent damage to the common peroneal nerve as it winds over the fibula will result in 'foot drop' where there is inability to evert and dorsiflex the foot. The subject then has to walk with a high step so that the toes do not hit the ground prematurely and trip them up.

The vascular supply to the leg and foot is very important clinically. Frequently there is an impaired blood supply which leads to changes in the skin, pain in the muscles on walking and eventually death of the tissues (gangrene). It is therefore important to be able to palpate the normal pulses of the femoral artery, the popliteal and dorsalis pedis in the normal limb. Often the blockage is high in the aorta or iliacs, but sometimes it is limited to the leg arteries themselves. These blockages can often be removed or by-passed.

The venous return from the leg is also important, much more so from the clinical point of view than that of the upper limb! Varicose veins are abnormally dilated veins in the leg. The trouble lies in the functionless valves at the regions of the perforators at the ankles and at the perforating terminations of the great and small saphenous veins. Blood accumulates in the superficial veins, which are not equipped to deal with it. The veins dilate and the circulation in the subcutaneous tissues and skin suffers. In the case of the perforators on the medial side of the ankle this often results in discolouration of the skin and eventually to an ulcer.

A congenital abnormality is sometimes seen in the joints of the ankle which gives rise to a condition called **club foot**. In this condition the baby's foot is **plantarflexed** at the ankle, **inverted** and **adducted** in the foot. At birth many of the abnormalities lie in the soft tissues and can therefore be corrected by manipulation. However, if neglected, the bones ossify in an abnormal shape and the ligaments and capsules contract further. More drastic surgery is then required (the same story as with congenital dislocation of the hip). In describing these deformities certain terms are used. The abnormal plantarflexed ankle is called the position of **equinus**. The abnormal position in which the foot points towards the midline is called **varus**. The generic name for an abnormal position in the ankle region is **talipes**; therefore the condition is called **talipes equinovarus**.

chapter 12

Summary and Revision of the Lower Limb

First use Figures 12.1, 12.2, 12.3 and 12.4 to revise both the course and distribution of the major nerves and the nerve supply to each of the muscles of the lower limb. Next read through the brief summaries of each muscle in each region of the lower limb. **Remember, do not try to learn origins and insertions in too much detail**. Concentrate on understanding each muscle and what it does as you read through the summaries. The small muscles of the foot are not included here since there is little merit in remembering details about them. A few key ligaments in the foot, however, have been included for revision purposes. Try not to learn the origins and insertions of muscles or the root values of nerves by heart but,

rather, concentrate on understanding general principles while you read these lists through. Finally, to bring together what you have learned, go through the multiple choice questions at the end of this chapter. For each **stem** any one of the five options (A–E) may be either correct or incorrect. Once again, some of the multiple choice questions in this section are difficult. On your first attempt at these questions a score of around 50% correct would be quite good. We expect you to have to refer back to the text to work out some of the answers and so improve your score when you attempt the questions again at a later date. As you do this, you will, of course, also improve your understanding of lower limb anatomy.

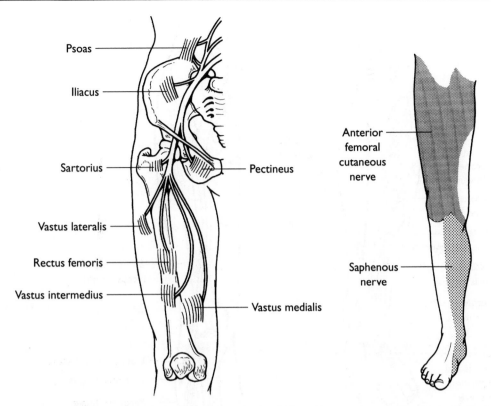

Figure 12.1 The course and distribution of the femoral nerve in the thigh and its cutaneous distribution in the leg (after Hollinshead, WH (1982) *Anatomy for Surgeons* 3rd edn. Philadelphia: Harper and Row).

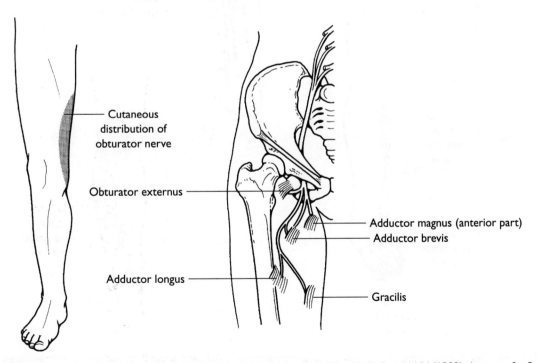

Figure 12.2 The course and distribution of the obturator nerve in the thigh (after Hollinshead, WH (1982) *Anatomy for Surgeons*, 3rd edn. Philadelphia: Harper and Row). Note that the obturator nerve has a cutaneous distribution on the medial aspect of the thigh.

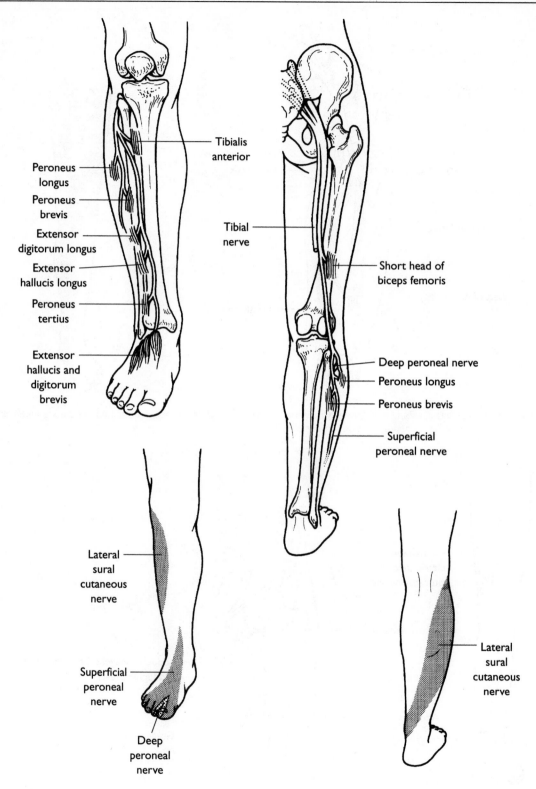

Figure 12.3   The course and distribution of the common peroneal nerve in the back of the thigh and leg (after Hollinshead, WH (1982) *Anatomy for Surgeons*, 3rd edn. Philadelphia: Harper and Row). The cutaneous distribution of the common peroneal nerve is also shown.

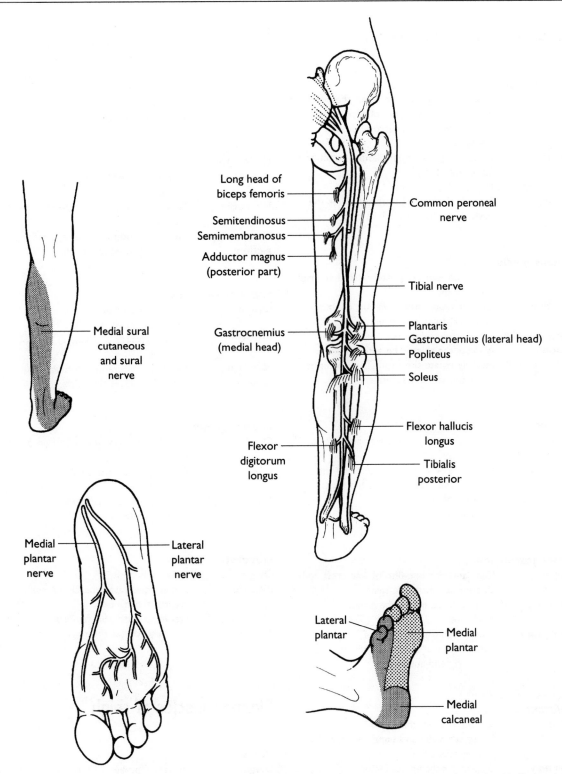

Long head of
biceps femoris

Semitendinosus

Semimembranosus

Adductor magnus
(posterior part)

Common peroneal
nerve

Tibial nerve

Plantaris
Gastrocnemius (lateral head)
Popliteus

Soleus

Gastrocnemius
(medial head)

Flexor hallucis
longus

Tibialis
posterior

Flexor
digitorum
longus

Medial sural
cutaneous
and sural
nerve

Medial
plantar
nerve

Lateral
plantar
nerve

Lateral
plantar

Medial
plantar

Medial
calcaneal

Figure 12.4   The course and distribution of the tibial nerve in the back of the thigh, the leg and foot (after Hollinshead, WH (1982) *Anatomy for Surgeons*, 3rd edn. Philadelphia: Harper and Row). Details of muscle innervation in the foot are omitted here. The cutaneous distribution of the tibial nerve is also shown.

Muscles of the gluteal region

Gluteus maximus
Origin: Ilium, between iliac crest and the posterior gluteal line. Lower part of sacrum, upper part of coccyx, and sacrotuberous ligament.
Insertion: Gluteal ridge of femur, iliotibial tract and fascia lata of thigh.
Nerve supply: Inferior gluteal nerve.
Action: Extends the thigh. Laterally rotates the thigh. Tightens the iliotibial tract.

Gluteus medius
Origin: Ilium, between the posterior and anterior gluteal lines.
Insertion: Greater trochanter of femur; oblique ridge on lateral surface of femur.
Nerve supply: Superior gluteal nerve.
Action: Abducts the thigh. The anterior fibres also medially rotate the thigh. The posterior fibres can laterally rotate the thigh.

Gluteus minimus
Origin: Ilium, between the anterior and inferior gluteal lines.
Insertion: Greater trochanter of femur at front, close to the capsule of the hip joint.
Nerve supply: Superior gluteal nerve.
Action: Abducts the thigh.

Tensor fasciae latae
Origin: Ilium, anterior one-fifth of iliac crest and anterior superior iliac spine.
Insertion: Iliotibial tract, below the greater trochanter.
Nerve supply: Superior gluteal nerve.
Action: Tenses the iliotibial tract. Pulls it superiorly and anteriorly.

Piriformis
Origin: Sacrum; second, third, and fourth segments and upper border of greater sciatic notch.
Insertion: Greater trochanter of femur (highest point).
Nerve supply: Sacral nerves 1 and 2.
Action: Laterally rotates the thigh.

Obturator externus
Origin: Obturator membrane (medial half of outer surface) and from the adjacent pubis (body and inferior ramus) and ischium (ramus).
Insertion: Femur (trochanteric fossa).
Nerve supply: Obturator nerve (L2, 3, 4).
Action: Laterally rotates the thigh.

Obturator internus
Origin: Obturator membrane (lateral half of inner surface).
Insertion: Femur (inner surface of greater trochanter).
Nerve supply: Nerve to obturator internus (L5; S1, 2).
Action: Laterally rotates the thigh.

Superior gemellus
Origin: Ischial spine (upper margin of lesser sciatic notch).
Insertion: Femur (greater trochanter) with obturator internus.
Nerve supply: Nerve to obturator internus.
Action: Laterally rotates the thigh.

Inferior gemellus
Origin: Ischial tuberosity (lower margin of lesser sciatic notch).
Insertion: Femur (greater trochanter) with obturator internus.
Nerve supply: Nerve to quadratus femoris.
Action: Laterally rotates the thigh.

Quadratus femoris
Origin: Ischial tuberosity.
Insertion: Femur (quadrate tubercle on back of greater trochanter).
Nerve supply: Nerve to quadratus femoris.
Action: Laterally rotates the thigh.

Flexor muscles of thigh

Psoas
Origin: Vertebral bodies T12–L5.
Insertion: Lesser trochanter of femur.
Nerve supply: L2 and 3.
Action: Flexes the thigh and medially rotates it.

Iliacus

Origin: Iliac fossa and sacrum.
Insertion: Into the tendon of psoas and then to lesser trochanter of femur.
Nerve supply: L2 and 3.
Action: Flexes the thigh.

Adductors of the thigh

Adductor longus

Origin: From the pubis immediately below pubic crest.
Insertion: Linea aspera of femur.
Nerve supply: Obturator nerve (L2, 3, 4) anterior division.
Action: Adducts thigh. It is also a lateral rotator and can flex the extended thigh.

Pectineus

Origin: From the pubis.
Insertion: Upper half of line running from lesser trochanter to linea aspera of femur.
Nerve supply: Femoral nerve (occasionally obturator nerve).
Action: Adducts the thigh. It also has a flexor action.

Adductor magnus

Origin: Ischial tuberosity and inferior pubic ramus.
Insertion: Femur; a line running from greater trochanter, along linea aspera to the adductor tubercle of the femur.
Nerve supply: Obturator nerve (posterior division) and sciatic nerve.
Action: Adducts thigh. The posterior part of the muscle extends the thigh.

Gracilis

Origin: Body and inferior ramus of pubis.
Insertion: Upper part of medial surface of tibia.
Nerve supply: Obturator nerve (anterior division).
Action: Adducts thigh. Flexes the knee joint. Medially rotates the leg.

Adductor brevis

Origin: Pubis; outer surface of body and inferior ramus.
Insertion: Femur; line running from lesser trochanter to linea aspera, and upper part of linea aspera.
Nerve supply: Obturator nerve.
Action: Adducts the thigh.

Extensors of the knee, flexors of the hip

Rectus femoris

Origin: Anterior inferior iliac spine.
Insertion: Patella; via tendon, then via patellar ligament to tibial tuberosity.
Nerve supply: Femoral nerve (L2, 3, 4).
Action: Extends the leg. Flexes the thigh.

Vastus lateralis

Origin: Femur; intertrochanteric line, linea aspera and lateral supracondylar line.
Insertion: Tibial tuberosity via patella.
Nerve supply: Femoral nerve (L2, 3, 4).
Action: Extends the leg.

Vastus medialis

Origin: Femur; anterior intertrochanteric line, linea aspera and medial epicondylar line.
Insertion: Tibial tuberosity via patellar ligament.
Nerve supply: Femoral nerve (L2, 3, 4).
Action: Extends the leg.

Vastus intermedius

Origin: Femur; anterior and lateral surfaces.
Insertion: Tibial tuberosity via patella.
Nerve supply: Femoral nerve (L2, 3).
Action: Extends the leg.

Flexors of the knee, extensors of the hip

Sartorius

Origin: Anterior superior iliac spine.
Insertion: Upper part of medial surface of tibia.
Nerve supply: Femoral nerve.
Action: Flexes the thigh. Flexes the leg. Laterally rotates the thigh.

Biceps femoris

Origin: Long head from ischial tuberosity of pelvis. Short head from lower part of linea aspera.
Insertion: Head of fibula.
Nerve supply: Sciatic nerve or common peroneal nerve.
Action: Flexes the knee. Extends the hip.

Semitendinosus
Origin:	Ischial tuberosity.
Insertion:	Medial surface of shaft of tibia superiorly.
Nerve supply:	Sciatic nerve.
Action:	Flexes the knee. Extends the hip. Medial rotator of flexed knee.

Semimembranosus
Origin:	Ischial tuberosity.
Insertion:	Tibia. Groove at back of medial condyle.
Nerve supply:	Sciatic nerve.
Action:	Flexes the knee. Extends the hip. Medial rotator of flexed knee.

Popliteus
Origin:	Femur, lateral condyle inside capsule of knee joint.
Insertion:	Tibia, popliteal line on posterior surface.
Nerve supply:	Tibial nerve.
Action:	Unlocks knee by laterally rotating the femur. Can flex knee joint weakly.

The anterior group of leg muscles

Tibialis anterior
Origin:	Tibia, upper half of lateral surface.
Insertion:	Medial side of medial cuneiform and first metatarsal.
Nerve supply:	Deep peroneal nerve.
Action:	Dorsiflexes the ankle. Inverts the foot.

Extensor digitorum longus
Origin:	Fibula, upper three-quarters of anterior surface and intermuscular septum.
Insertion:	Middle and distal phalanges of lateral four toes.
Nerve supply:	Deep peroneal nerve.
Action:	Extends the interphalangeal and metatarsophalangeal joints of toes and dorsiflexes the foot.

Extensor hallucis
Origin:	Fibula, middle of anterior surface.
Insertion:	Great toe; terminal phalanx.
Nerve supply:	Deep peroneal nerve.
Action:	Extends the great toe. Dorsiflexes the ankle.

Peroneus longus
Origin:	Fibula, upper two-thirds of lateral aspect.
Insertion:	Lateral aspect of medial cuneiform and base of first metatarsal.
Nerve supply:	Superficial peroneal nerve.
Action:	Everts the foot. Plantarflexes the ankle joint.

Peroneus brevis
Origin:	Fibula, lower two-thirds of lateral aspect.
Insertion:	5th metatarsal, peroneal tubercle.
Nerve supply:	Superficial peroneal nerve.
Action:	Everts the foot. Plantarflexes the ankle joint.

Peroneus tertius
Origin:	Fibula, lower quarter and anterior surface.
Insertion:	Shaft of 5th metatarsal.
Nerve supply:	Deep peroneal nerve.
Action:	Everts the foot. Dorsiflexes the ankle.

The posterior group of leg muscles

Gastrocnemius
Origin:	Lateral head from lateral epicondyle and lateral supracondylar line of femur; medial head from surface of femur above medial epicondyle.
Insertion:	Via tendo calcaneus into calcaneus.
Nerve supply:	Tibial nerve.
Action:	Plantarflexes ankle joint. Flexes knee joint.

Soleus
Origin:	From back of head and upper third of shaft of fibula and from middle third of medial border of tibia. A fibrous arch joins these two origins.
Insertion:	With gastrocnemius via tendo calcaneus into the calcaneus.
Nerve supply:	Tibial nerve.
Action:	Plantarflexes ankle joint.

Plantaris
Origin:	From lateral epicondyle of femur.
Insertion:	Into the tendo calcaneus.
Nerve supply:	Tibial nerve.
Action:	Weak plantarflexor of foot at ankle joint.

Tibialis posterior

Origin: Interosseous membrane and from back of head and upper two-thirds of fibula and medial surface of shaft and from lateral aspect of tibia.

Insertion: Tuberosity of navicular. Medial cuneiform with slips to other tarsal bones (except talus) as well as to 2nd, 3rd and 4th metatarsals.

Nerve supply: Tibial nerve.

Action: Plantar flexes ankle joint. Inverts foot.

Flexor digitorum longus

Origin: From tibia, posterior surface medial to vertical line.

Insertion: Each tendon passes through the tendon of flexor digitorum brevis to be inserted into the distal phalanx of toes 2–5.

Nerve supply: Tibial nerve.

Action: Flexes phalanges of toes. Maintains longitudinal arches of foot.

Flexor hallucis longus

Origin: From fibula, lower two-thirds of posterior surface.

Insertion: Base of distal phalanx of great toe.

Nerve supply: Tibial nerve.

Action: Flexes phalanges of great toe.

Important Ligaments in the Foot

The 'spring ligament' or plantar calcaneonavicular ligament

This ligament bridges the gap between the sustentaculum tali and the navicular bone on the plantar aspect of the talocalcaneonavicular joint. It lies beneath the head of the talus.

The short plantar ligament

The short plantar ligament consists of a thick bundle of fibres that run from the anterior tubercle on the front of the undersurface of the calcaneum to the cuboid bone in front of it.

The long plantar ligament

The long plantar ligament overlies the short plantar ligament. It arises from further back on the calcaneus, from the posterior tubercles, runs forwards over the anterior tubercle and bridges a groove on the cuboid (for the tendon of the peroneus longus). It then extends further forwards to the heads of the central three metatarsal bones.

Multiple Choice Questions On The Lower Limb

1. Concerning movements at the hip joint:
(A) flexion may be produced by the iliopsoas
(B) extension may be produced by the hamstring muscles
(C) lateral rotation may be produced by the piriformis
(D) medial rotation may be produced by the tensor fasciae latae
(E) extension is limited by the iliofemoral ligament

A＿＿ B ＿＿ C ＿＿ D ＿＿ E ＿＿

2. The obturator internus:
(A) forms the floor of the pelvic cavity
(B) arises from the obturator membrane
(C) is covered with strong fascia on its pelvic surface
(D) inserts into the lesser trochanter
(E) is a lateral rotator of the thigh at the hip joint

A＿＿ B ＿＿ C ＿＿ D ＿＿ E ＿＿

3. The femoral nerve:
(A) lies in the groove between iliacus and psoas muscles
(B) is a branch of the lumbar plexus
(C) passes through the adductor canal
(D) supplies motor fibres to the quadratus femoris muscle
(E) has a branch called the lateral femoral cutaneous nerve of the thigh

A＿＿ B ＿＿ C ＿＿ D ＿＿ E ＿＿

4. Superficial inguinal lymph nodes receive lymph:
(A) from the abdominal wall
(B) from the testes
(C) from the lower anal canal
(D) from the bladder
(E) from the lower limb

A＿＿ B ＿＿ C ＿＿ D ＿＿ E ＿＿

5. Muscles that can produce lateral rotation at the hip joint are:
(A) piriformis
(B) tensor fasciae latae
(C) quadratus femoris
(D) gracilis
(E) sartorius

A＿＿ B ＿＿ C ＿＿ D ＿＿ E ＿＿

6. Muscles that insert into the greater trochanter include:
(A) psoas
(B) gluteus medius
(C) gluteus maximus
(D) piriformis
(E) tensor fasciae latae

A＿＿ B ＿＿ C ＿＿ D ＿＿ E ＿＿

7. The saphenous opening:
(A) transmits the small saphenous vein
(B) transmits the saphenous nerve
(C) is a defect in the femoral sheath
(D) may transmit a femoral hernia
(E) has a falciform edge

A＿＿ B ＿＿ C ＿＿ D ＿＿ E ＿＿

8. Boundaries of the femoral ring include:
(A) the inguinal ligament
(B) the femoral artery
(C) the inferior pubic ramus
(D) the pectineal ligament
(E) the lacunar ligament

A＿＿ B ＿＿ C ＿＿ D ＿＿ E ＿＿

9. Contents of the femoral canal include:
(A) the femoral vein
(B) a lymph node
(C) fat
(D) the femoral nerve
(E) lymphatics

A＿＿ B ＿＿ C ＿＿ D ＿＿ E ＿＿

10. With regard to the femur:
(A) part of biceps femoris takes origin from the femoral shaft
(B) the iliofemoral ligament attaches to the intertrochanteric line
(C) there is a synovial joint between the femur and the fibula at the knee
(D) the head of the femur begins to ossify before birth
(E) rectus femoris takes origin from the femoral shaft

A＿＿ B ＿＿ C ＿＿ D ＿＿ E ＿＿

11. Gluteus maximus:
(A) arises from the iliac tubercle on the iliac crest
(B) is inserted into the iliotibial tract and femur
(C) is supplied by a branch of the sciatic nerve
(D) extends the trunk on the thigh when rising from the sitting position
(E) aids in medial rotation at the hip joint

A＿＿ B ＿＿ C ＿＿ D ＿＿ E ＿＿

12. The psoas major muscle:
(A) arises from spinous processes of all the lumbar vertebrae
(B) inserts into the lesser trochanter
(C) is enclosed in a fibrous sheath
(D) is innervated by the lumbar plexus
(E) is a flexor of the hip joint

A＿＿ B ＿＿ C ＿＿ D ＿＿ E ＿＿

13. The sartorius muscle:
(A) is attached to the anterior inferior iliac spine
(B) forms one boundary of the femoral triangle
(C) rotates the hip laterally
(D) is attached distally to the medial femoral condyle
(E) is supplied by the obturator nerve

A＿＿ B ＿＿ C ＿＿ D ＿＿ E ＿＿

14. The greater sciatic foramen:
(A) transmits the superior gluteal nerve
(B) transmits the obturator internus muscle
(C) transmits the pudendal nerve
(D) has the sacrospinous ligament as a boundary
(E) transmits the internal pudendal artery

A___ B___ C___ D___ E___

15. The piriformis muscle:
(A) arises within the pelvic cavity
(B) has the internal pudendal artery at its upper border
(C) rotates the thigh laterally
(D) has the sciatic nerve at its lower border
(E) inserts on the lesser trochanter of the femur

A___ B___ C___ D___ E___

16. Contents of the adductor canal include:
(A) the long saphenous vein
(B) the femoral artery
(C) the saphenous nerve
(D) the profunda femoris artery
(E) the nerve to vastus medialis

A___ B___ C___ D___ E___

17. The obturator nerve:
(A) is a motor nerve only
(B) leaves the pelvis beneath the lateral part of the inguinal ligament
(C) innervates the obturator externus muscle
(D) innervates the obturator internus muscle
(E) is found in the adductor canal

A___ B___ C___ D___ E___

18. The tibial nerve:
(A) has a segmental composition L2–L4
(B) innervates the long head of the biceps femoris muscle
(C) passes through the popliteal fossa superficial to the popliteal vein
(D) supplies both heads of the gastrocnemius muscle
(E) ends by dividing into the medial and lateral plantar nerves

A___ B___ C___ D___ E___

19. The profunda femoris artery:
(A) is a direct branch of the external iliac artery
(B) gives off the inferior gluteal artery
(C) gives rise to perforating arteries which supply the adductor muscles of the thigh
(D) contributes to the cruciform anastomosis
(E) becomes the popliteal artery at the adductor hiatus

A___ B___ C___ D___ E___

20. The anterior cruciate ligament of the knee:
(A) attaches to the medial condyle of the femur
(B) is completely surrounded by synovial membrane
(C) attaches to the anterior part of the intercondylar area of the tibia
(D) transmits blood vessels
(E) is taut when standing with the weight taken on a flexed knee

A___ B___ C___ D___ E___

21. With respect to the knee:
(A) the lateral meniscus is firmly adherent to the lateral collateral ligament
(B) the popliteus tendon runs through the joint cavity
(C) the suprapatella bursa communicates with the joint capsule
(D) the medial tibial condyle is smaller than the lateral
(E) the posterior cruciate ligament is taut in hyperflexion

A___ B___ C___ D___ E___

22. Gastrocnemius:
(A) has three heads of origin
(B) arises from the tibia
(C) inserts into the calcaneus
(D) is supplied by the common peroneal nerve
(E) is an evertor of the foot at the ankle

A___ B___ C___ D___ E___

23. The patella:
(A) is a sesamoid bone
(B) articulates with the tibia
(C) is attached to the tibia by the ligamentum patellae
(D) has a bursa between itself and the skin
(E) has its deep surface completely covered by synovial membrane

A___ B___ C___ D___ E___

24. The popliteal artery:
(A) lies against the posterior surface of the femur
(B) ends by dividing into anterior and posterior tibial arteries
(C) lies superficial (posterior) to the popliteal vein in the fossa
(D) gives genicular branches
(E) lies on the posterior surface of the popliteus muscle

A___ B___ C___ D___ E___

25. The great saphenous vein:
(A) is accompanied in the leg by the sural nerve
(B) receives blood from veins in the soleus
(C) passes over the anterior surface of the medial malleolus
(D) passes through the saphenous opening
(E) contains no valves

A___ B___ C___ D___ E___

26. Extensor hallucis longus:
(A) is supplied by the superficial peroneal nerve
(B) everts the foot
(C) dorsiflexes the big toe
(D) has its tendon on the medial side of the dorsalis pedis artery
(E) can dorsiflex the foot at the ankle joint

A___ B___ C___ D___ E___

27. The deep peroneal nerve:
(A) supplies tibialis anterior
(B) supplies skin over the front of the lateral malleolus
(C) supplies peroneus longus
(D) supplies extensor digitorum longus
(E) supplies peroneus tertius

A___ B___ C___ D___ E___

28. Peroneus longus:
(A) arises from the fibula
(B) passes deep to two peroneal retinacula
(C) creates a groove on the cuboid bone
(D) inserts into the base of the 5th metatarsal
(E) is supplied by the superficial peroneal nerve

A___ B ___ C ___ D ___ E ___

29. Structures passing deep to the flexor retinaculum at the ankle include:
(A) peroneus longus tendon
(B) tibial nerve
(C) tibialis anterior tendon
(D) flexor hallucis longus tendon
(E) deep peroneal nerve

A___ B ___ C ___ D ___ E ___

30. With respect to the foot:
(A) the dorsalis pedis artery lies between the tendons of tibialis anterior and extensor hallucis longus
(B) the deep peroneal nerve supplies sensation to the web of skin between the great and second toe
(C) the long plantar ligament runs between the calcaneus and the navicular
(D) the tibialis posterior tendon passes deep to the deltoid ligament
(E) peroneus brevis inserts into the peroneal tubercle of the 5th metatarsal

A___ B ___ C ___ D ___ E ___

Answers to Multiple Choice Questions

1.	A T	B T	C T	D T	E T
2.	A F	B T	C T	D F	E T
3.	A T	B T	C F	D F	E F
4.	A T	B F	C T	D F	E T
5.	A T	B F	C T	D F	E T
6.	A F	B T	C F	D T	E F
7.	A F	B F	C F	D T	E T
8.	A T	B F	C F	D T	E T
9.	A F	B T	C T	D F	E T
10.	A T	B T	C F	D F	E F

11.	A F	B T	C F	D T	E F
12.	A F	B T	C T	D T	E T
13.	A F	B T	C T	D F	E F
14.	A T	B F	C T	D T	E T
15.	A T	B F	C T	D T	E F
16.	A F	B T	C T	D F	E T
17.	A F	B F	C T	D F	E F
18.	A F	B T	C T	D T	E T
19.	A F	B F	C T	D T	E F
20.	A F	B F	C T	D F	E F

21.	A F	B T	C T	D F	E T
22.	A F	B F	C T	D F	E F
23.	A T	B F	C T	D T	E F
24.	A T	B T	C F	D T	E T
25.	A F	B F	C T	D T	E F
26.	A F	B F	C T	D T	E T
27.	A T	B F	C F	D T	E T
28.	A T	B T	C T	D F	E T
29.	A F	B T	C F	D T	E F
30.	A T	B T	C F	D F	E T

THE VERTEBRAL COLUMN

The Vertebral Column

The vertebral column, rib cage and skull form the **axial skeleton**. The vertebral column supports the skull above, provides anchorage for the ribs, and protects the spinal cord. It is flexible and strong. Each bone in the vertebral column is called a **vertebra**. In the **cervical region** there are seven vertebrae, in the **thoracic region** there are 12 and in the **lumbar region** five. There are five fused sacral vertebral segments which are wedged between the two sides of the pelvis. The lower extremity of the column is composed of several small fused bones called the **coccyx**. Great strength is required to transmit the body weight through the column without it collapsing. Vertebrae are therefore stout. This is especially true in the lower parts of the column. The vertebral column is held together by a series of strong ligaments and muscles which move and support the vertebrae.

In infants the vertebral column is flexed like a letter 'C'. This anterior flexure is called the **primary curvature** (Fig. 13.1). During development two secondary curvatures develop in the cervical and lumbar regions (Fig. 13.2). The **secondary cervical curvature** develops as children begin to hold their head up along with the development of the muscular support needed to balance the head. The centre of gravity in the head is such that it tends to flex forwards on to the chest when unsupported. Strong extensor muscles develop at the back of the neck to counter this. The **secondary lumbar curvature** develops as children learn to walk upright and balance on two feet. Both the cervical and lumbar curvatures are concave posteriorly.

Lordosis is an increased anterior convexity of the vertebral column and is commonly seen in the lumbar region. **Kyphosis** means the opposite, an increase in the posterior convexity of the spine. **Scoliosis** is a lateral curvature and rotational deformity, and often occurs together with either lordosis or kyphosis.

Thoracic vertebrae

Vertebrae differ in shape from region to region. None the less, a basic pattern does exist and this is seen most clearly by studying the **thoracic vertebrae** first. Each thoracic vertebra is composed of two basic parts. Anteriorly there is a mass of bone called the **body**. Posteriorly there is a crescent of bone called the **vertebral arch**. Body and arch together enclose a hole, the **vertebral foramen** (Fig. 13.3). Three bony processes arise from the vertebral arch. These give attachment to muscles and ligaments. They are called the **spinous process** and the right and left **transverse processes**. The spinous process projects backwards and downwards from the middle of the vertebral arch, and the transverse processes project sideways from either side. The transverse processes divide the vertebral arch into two parts. That part lying between the body and process is called the **pedicle**, and the rest is the **lamina**. It is the laminae, therefore, that bear the spinous process. Each thoracic vertebra articulates with a pair of ribs (Fig. 13.4). In fact vertebrae in the cervical and lumbar region also have a 'costal element' which represents an undeveloped rib. Sometimes these elements are well developed, giving rise to **cervical** or **lumbar ribs**. On the lateral aspects of the bodies of all but the first (T1) and last two (T11 and T12) thoracic vertebrae, there are hemifacets at

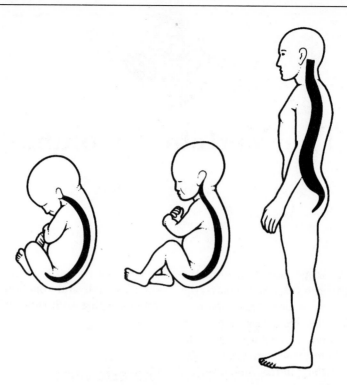

Figure 13.1 Development of the secondary cervical and lumbar curvatures of the spine occurs as the head is supported and with upright posture.

the top and bottom for articulation with the ribs. Each rib articulates with the vertebra of its own number and also with the one above. The head of the rib therefore straddles the intervertebral disc in between the vertebral bodies. Ribs at T1, T11 and T12 articulate only with the thoracic vertebra of their own number. Ribs also articulate with the transverse processes of their own thoracic vertebrae at another synovial joint.

The 12 thoracic vertebrae sit one on top of the other. In so doing, the vertebral foramina form one continuous tube called the **vertebral canal**. This contains the spinal cord. Between each pair of vertebrae, however, there is an exit on the right and the left side from the vertebral canal. These openings allow spinal nerves, arteries and veins to pass in and out of the canal. These are called **intervertebral foramina** (Fig. 13.5). Vertebrae articulate with one another by means of joints. They are further joined by ligaments. Basically there are two articulations between any pair of vertebrae, **body to body** and **vertebral arch to vertebral arch**.

The body of one vertebra articulates with the body of another by means of a **secondary cartilaginous**

joint called an **intervertebral disc**. Covering the surface of each vertebral body in the region of the disc is a thin layer of cartilage. Uniting these cartilages is a mesh of strong fibrous tissue that can withstand strains in any direction during movements of one body on another. However, since the fibrous tissue exists only around the periphery of the disc, it is called the **annulus fibrosus** (Fig. 13.6). The centre of the disc is not fibrous. It consists of a gelatinous 'ball' called the **nucleus pulposus** (Fig. 13.7). The bodies of the vertebrae can move around this central mass in any direction. Theoretically, if these were the only articulations between vertebrae, the column would be freely movable in all directions. Notice the relationship of the disc to the vertebral canal and intervertebral foramen. Degeneration sometimes occurs in the disc. The nucleus pulposus can then herniate through a split in the posterior surface of the annulus. If this occurs the spinal cord or a spinal nerve can be compressed, resulting in various neurological symptoms. This condition is called a **herniated intervertebral disc**, or more commonly a 'slipped disc' (Fig. 13.8).

Vertebral bodies are also held together by longitudinal ligaments. The **anterior longitudinal ligament**

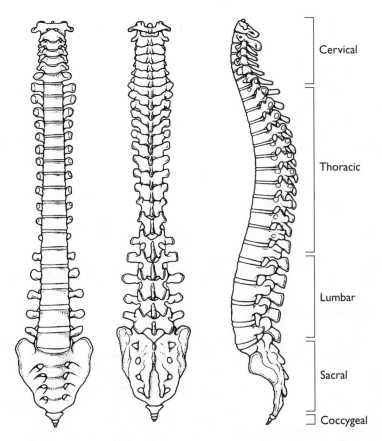

Figure 13.2   The vertebral column is made up of cervical, thoracic, lumbar, sacral and coccygeal regions. The individual vertebrae in each region are distinct but there is also a gradual change in morphology from one region to the next.

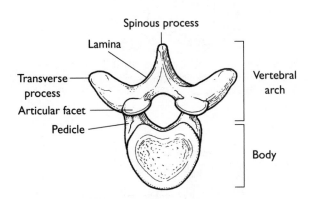

Figure 13.3   The component parts of a typical thoracic vertebra.

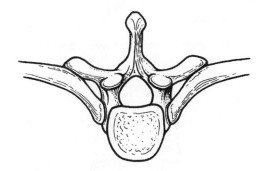

Figure 13.4   Both the head and tubercle of a rib articulate with thoracic vertebrae at synovial joints.

extends from the cervical region to the sacrum, uniting the anterior surfaces of the bodies. It is not attached to the intervertebral discs (Fig. 13.9). The **posterior longitudinal ligament** on the other hand extends from vertebra to vertebra in the vertebral canal behind the bodies. This ligament *is* attached to each intervertebral disc and is narrow over each body (Fig. 13.10).

The **vertebral arches** also articulate one with the other. These articulations are **synovial joints**. Each vertebral arch bears four **articular facets**. Two are for

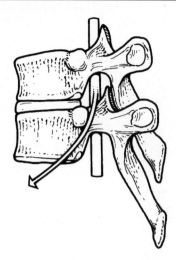

Figure 13.5   An intervertebral foramen is bounded in front by the bodies and intervertebral disc, above and below by the pedicles, and posteriorly by the synovial facet joints between the vertebral arches of the vertebrae above and below. Spinal nerves and vessels pass through the intervertebral foramina.

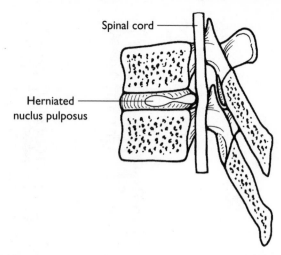

Figure 13.8   With a herniated or prolapsed intervertebral disc, the nucleus pulposus protrudes through the annulus fibrosus and may impinge on the spinal cord or spinal nerves within the vertebral canal.

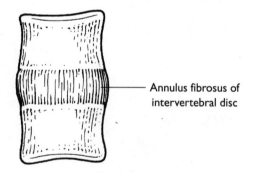

Figure 13.6   Vertebral bodies are joined together by intervertebral discs which are secondary cartilaginous joints.

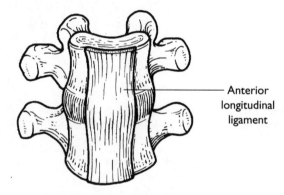

Figure 13.9   The anterior longitudinal ligament unites the anterior surfaces of the vertebral bodies but does not attach to the intervertebral discs.

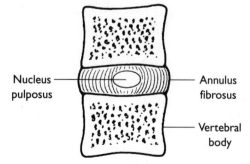

Figure 13.7   In a section through an intervertebral disc the annulus fibrosus and the nucleus pulposus can be identified.

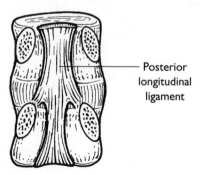

Figure 13.10   The posterior longitudinal ligament attaches to both the vertebral bodies and the intervertebral discs.

articulation with the vertebra above and two for the vertebra below. The **plane** at which these articular facets are set varies with the region of the column. The plane of movement in these joints therefore limits the 'universal' movement that would be permitted by the body to body articulation alone. Notice that in the thoracic region the facets lie on the arc of a circle (Fig. 13.11). The centre of this circle is usually near to the nucleus pulposus (but not consistently so). Movements of flexion are therefore limited; the articular facets allow mostly a rotational movement between the vertebrae in this region. In fact, even this movement is not very great, since the ribs in the thoracic region also limit movements between the thoracic vertebrae.

Several **ligaments** also attach the vertebral arches together. The **ligamenta flava** are yellow elastic ligaments that bind adjacent laminae together (Fig. 13.12). The processes of the vertebral arches are also bounded by ligaments. The **supraspinous** and **interspinous** ligaments bind the spinous processes together. The supraspinous ligaments bind the tips and the interspinous ligaments the bodies of the spinous processes. The **intertransverse ligaments** join the transverse processes to one another.

The thoracic vertebrae are not easy to see on a radiograph. They are always obscured to some extent by the ribs. The usual views taken of vertebrae are **lateral** and **anteroposterior**. On a lateral radiograph the various parts can easily be identified. The intervertebral foramina are easily seen in lateral view (Fig. 13.13) but are, however, shown a little clearer if a slightly oblique view is taken.

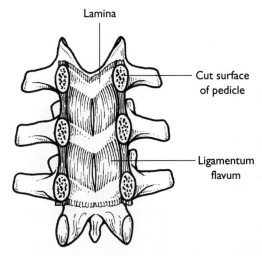

Figure 13.12 The ligamentum flavum is an elastic ligament which is attached between adjacent lamina. Here, the pedicles have been cut and the vertebral bodies removed to show the ligamenta flava from within the vertebral canal. There is often a midline deficiency between the ligaments of each side.

Cervical vertebrae

The cervical vertebrae (Figs 13.14 and 13.15) are smaller and more delicate than thoracic vertebrae. They are seven in number. The first and second (**atlas** and **axis**) are very special, being adapted to support the skull and to allow the movements of nodding and rotation of the head respectively. Let us look first, however, at the 'typical' cervical vertebrae (C3–7), noting how they differ from the thoracic pattern.

The bodies of cervical vertebrae are small and

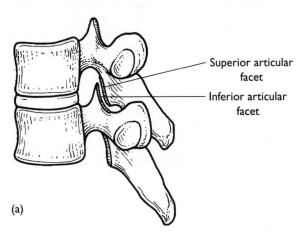

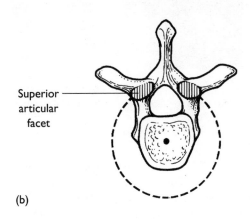

(a)

(b)

Figure 13.11 The facet joints between adjacent thoracic vertebrae are aligned to allow slight rotational movements between vertebrae.

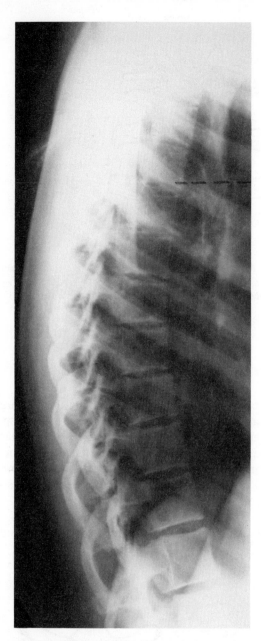

Figure 13.13 Identify the intervertebral foramina, the intervertebral discs and the facet joints in this lateral radiograph of the thorax. The dotted line lies at the level of the 4th thoracic vertebra and the manubriosternal joint.

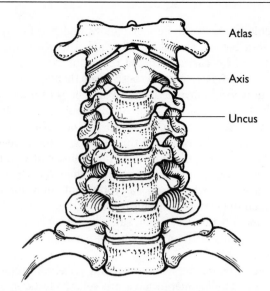

Figure 13.14 The altas and axis are atypical cervical vertebrae with special functions. Understand that there are seven cervical vertebrae and note the uncus, or upturned lip, on the bodies of the cervical vertebrae which form synovial uncovertebral joints between each pair of adjacent vertebrae.

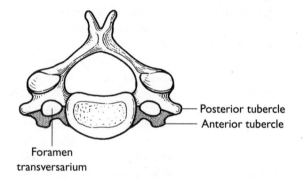

Figure 13.15 Seen from above, a typical cervical vertebrae has transverse processes, each with a foramen transversarium in it and with anterior and posterior tubercles at its lateral extremity. It also has a small oval-shaped body, a large triangular vertebral canal and a bifid spinous process. In this figure the costal element is stippled.

delicate and oval in shape when viewed from above (Fig. 13.15). They are joined together by intervertebral discs. These are strengthened by the anterior and posterior longitudinal ligaments. The vertebral arch together with the body encloses a vertebral foramen, which in this region is triangular in shape and very large, since the spinal cord is biggest in this region. The bodies of cervical vertebrae have small upturned lips on the upper lateral margins. Each one is called an **uncus** and they form **uncovertebral joints** between successive vertebral bodies. Uncovertebral joints occur only between cervical vertebrae and are associated with rotational movements of the cervical column. (Animals such as horses and cattle which sway their heads from side to side do not have them.)

The processes of the arch in cervical vertebrae

require special consideration. In the transverse processes of all cervical vertebrae there is a hole called the **foramen transversarium**. In the cervical column these foramina lie one above the other. Through these foramina, on either side, a branch of the subclavian artery ascends towards the skull. It is the **vertebral artery**. The right and left vertebral arteries enter the foramina transversaria of the 6th cervical vertebra. They eventually enter the skull through the foramen magnum where they help to supply the brain and spinal cord with arterial blood.

Anterior and **posterior tubercles** can be clearly seen on each transverse process. These give attachment to the scalenus anterior, scalenus medius and scalenus posterior muscles in the neck. In fact only the posterior tubercle belongs developmentally to the transverse process. The anterior tubercle is the degenerated cervical rib. It is the **costal element** of the cervical vertebra. Sometimes the anterior tubercle of the 7th vertebra is large and can even form a complete rib. We have noted that this extra rib is then called a 'cervical rib' (Fig. 13.16).

The **spinous processes** of the cervical vertebrae are bifid. All processes are united by ligaments, supraspinous and interspinous and intertransverse. The **vertebral arches** articulate with one another by means of articular processes. These joints are synovial. The facets do not lie on the arc of a circle as in the thoracic region. They therefore allow little rotation between individual typical cervical vertebrae. They lie almost in a coronal plane so that lateral flexion as well as flexion and extension are all permitted. As elsewhere the laminae are united by ligamenta flava. The articu-

lar facets between the vertebrae are also clearly seen in Figure 13.17.

The spinous process of C7 is the largest and most prominent of the cervical vertebrae. That is not to say that the uppermost thoracic vertebrae may not be even more prominent, but the spinous process of C7 is the first in the neck that can easily be seen and palpated. By counting down from this prominent spine it can be used to identify the spines of each vertebra below this level. The 7th cervical vertebra is therefore called the **vertebra prominens.**

The **atlas** and **axis** require special study. The atlas has no body. It is simply a ring of bone consisting of an **anterior arch** and a **posterior arch** united on either side by two **lateral masses** made up of transverse processes and articular facets. It is modified in this way for two reasons. It has to support the skull and it allows a nodding movement between its superior articular facets and the occipital condyles of the skull (Fig. 13.18).

Unlike the atlas, the axis does have a body, but on

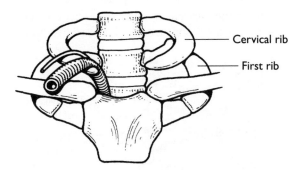

Figure 13.16 Rarely, the costal element of the last or 7th cervical vertebra develops into a so-called 'cervical rib'. This can often impede blood flow in the subclavian vessels and stretch the lower nerve roots of the brachial plexus, especially the contribution from T1. This can present first with weakness in the small muscles of the hand.

Cervical rib

First rib

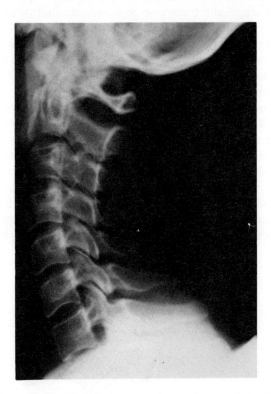

Figure 13.17 Note the large prominent spinous process of the 7th cervical vertebra and the angulation of the facet joints in this lateral radiograph of the neck. Try also to identify the position of the dens of the axis behind the anterior arch of the atlas. This is not always easy in this view.

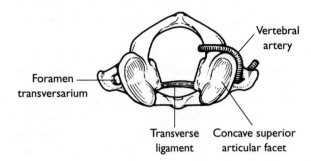

Figure 13.18 The atlas and the vertebral artery seen from above. Note the anterior arch of the atlas, the transverse ligament, and the concave superior articular facets that articulate with the occipital condyles.

top of it is a peg of bone called the **dens** or **odontoid process** of the axis (Fig. 13.19). This peg, in fact, is said to be the body of the atlas which has become attached to the axis. The function of the dens is to project into a socket within the ring of the atlas and so allow **rotation** of the atlas and head around itself.

Both atlas and axis have a foramen transversarium in each of the transverse processes, through which the vertebral arteries course. Having reached the foramen transversarium of the atlas, the vertebral artery curves back over the lateral mass of the atlas and its posterior arch to enter the vertebral canal and foramen magnum.

Look carefully at the joints between the atlas and skull and between the axis and atlas. The **superior articular facet** of the **atlas** is concave and kidney shaped (Fig. 13.18). Each facet accepts an occipital condyle at the base of the skull. The articulations are synovial and allow the facets to slide against one another. They allow only flexion and extension, that is a nodding type of movement of the head. A slight degree of side to side rocking is possible, but **no**

rotation. Now look at the articulation between atlas and axis. The **superior articular facets** on the axis lie at either side of the base of the dens (Fig. 13.19). They articulate with the inferior facets of the atlas. These synovial joints allow **only** rotation of the atlas ring on the axis around the dens. Their articular surfaces have to be flat to allow this. Strong ligaments stabilize all these joints (Fig. 13.20). Look into the vertebral canal from behind. First notice that the dens is inserted into a socket formed by the anterior arch of the atlas and a **transverse ligament**. This peg and socket joint is synovial. From the dens, three ligaments extend to the interior of the base of the skull. The transverse ligament is also continuous upwards and downwards as a sort of second layer of support. The upper continuation hides the three short ligaments and is attached to the skull while the lower extension is attached to the body of the axis. These four ligaments are collectively called the **cruciate ligament** (Fig. 13.21). On the posterior surface of all these ligaments the **posterior longitudinal ligament** is continued up into the base of the skull as a sort of third layer of support. In this region it is called the **membrana tectoria**. Thus the atlas is sandwiched between skull and axis and all these ligaments act to stabilize each of the articulations between the three bones. Radiographs of the atlas and axis are best taken through the open mouth on to an X-ray plate positioned at the back of the neck.

Lumbar vertebrae

Lumbar vertebrae are more massive and stronger than either the cervical or thoracic vertebrae. Their processes are short and strong. There are five lumbar

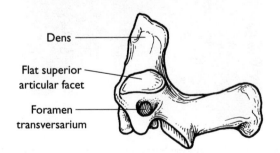

Figure 13.19 The superior articular facets of the axis are flat to allow rotation of the head. The dens is easily seen in this view as is the spinous process of the axis, which is quite large. Remember the atlas does not have a spinous process.

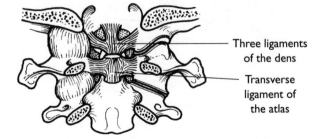

Figure 13.20 The apical and two lateral, or ala, ligaments of the dens pass to the margin of the occipital bone. The transverse ligament of the atlas holds the dens against the anterior arch of the atlas.

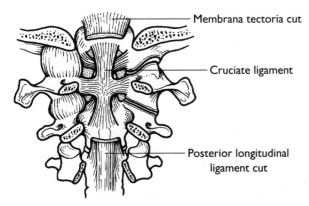

Membrana tectoria cut

Cruciate ligament

Posterior longitudinal ligament cut

Figure 13.21 The transverse ligament of the atlas is continued upwards to the skull and downwards to the axis forming the so-called cruciate ligament. Three small ligaments from the tip of the dens also pass up to the occipital bone (the central one, or apical ligament, is hidden here behind the cruciate ligament). All of these ligaments are covered by the posterior longitudinal ligament, which in the region of the skull base is called the membrana tectoria.

vertebrae, and each is composed of a large kidney-shaped body and vertebral arch (Fig. 13.22) which enclose a small vertebral canal. The bodies are large and strong and united to each other by intervertebral discs. It is in the region of T12–L1 and L4–L5 and L5–S1 that degeneration and herniation of the discs commonly occur. The vertebral arches bear massive transverse and spinous processes. The spinous processes are not as long as thoracic spinous processes and in the lumbar region they project directly backwards, whereas those in the thoracic region tend to project downwards and backwards more. The trans-

verse process is in reality a **costal element**. The true morphological transverse process is a small mass of bone at the base. Sometimes the 'transverse process' of the first lumbar vertebra is separate, being united to the body by a synovial joint. This is a **lumbar rib**, but is much rarer than a cervical rib.

Ligaments uniting arches and processes in the lumbar region are thick and strong. The articular facets form synovial articulations between the vertebral arches. The joints are aligned in the sagittal plane. It follows that they allow flexion and extension and some lateral flexion of the lumbar part of the column. They do not allow rotation though. Radiographs of the lumbar vertebrae give clear views of the various parts (Fig. 13.23).

The intervertebral foramina in the lumbar region are bounded by the body and intervertebral disc anteriorly, pedicles above and below, and synovial joint behind between the superior and inferior articular facets. The region of a lumbar vertebra between the superior articular process above and the inferior articular process below is known as the **pars interarticularis.** Traumatic fractures across the

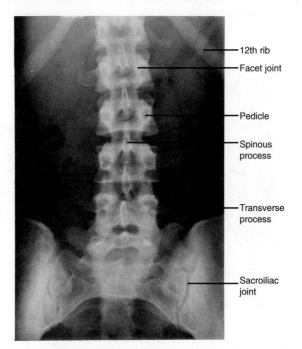

12th rib

Facet joint

Pedicle

Spinous process

Transverse process

Sacroiliac joint

Figure 13.23 The lumbar vertebral bodies gradually increase in width (along with the interpedicular distance) through the lumbar series. Note the various landmarks which are easily seen in this anteroposterior radiograph of the lumbar region. Count the lumbar vertebrae and look carefully at the last in this particular radiograph.

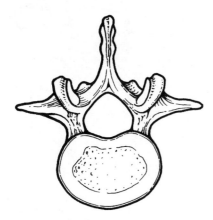

Figure 13.22 A lumbar vertebra seen from above has a large kidney-shaped body and facet joints which are oriented close to the sagittal plane. These allow anterior and posterior flexion and extension.

pars interarticularis are known as **spondylolysis.** On an oblique view of the lumbar vertebral column the pars can easily be recognized because it looks like the collar on a 'Scottie dog' (Fig. 13.24).   An abnormality that is sometimes seen in the 5th lumbar vertebra is called **spondylolisthesis.** Here there is failure of fusion between the body and arch during ossification. It's as if both collars of the 'Scottie dog' have failed to fuse. The body is then seen on a radiograph to have 'slipped' a little on the sacrum.

The sacrum and coccyx

The sacrum consists of five vertebrae that are fused to form one bony mass. However, the various parts of the vertebrae and their costal elements can still be recognized (Fig. 13.25). The sacrum is triangular in outline. Its upper surface articulates with the 5th lumbar vertebra by means of an intervertebral disc and by synovial joints between articular facets. On either side it articulates with the bones of the pelvis. The body weight does not pass through these joints, but through strong ligaments, **sacroiliac ligaments,** which join the bones. The **sacroiliac joints** are synovial joints. The anterior surface of the sacrum is con-

cave, but the first sacral mass bulges into the cavity of the pelvis. It is called the **promontory of the sacrum.** In the midline posteriorly, the fused vertebral bodies can be outlined by four transverse ridges of bone. These ridges represent the ossified intervertebral discs of the sacral region. On either side are four **anterior sacral foramina** through which the sacral ventral rami can pass. On each side of these foramina are two massive **lateral masses** of bone. These and the bone between them and the foramina represent the costal elements of the sacral vertebrae. The posterior surface of the sacrum is convex. In the midline posteriorly, the **median crest** is a ridge representing the fused spinous processes. In the midline below, the vertebral canal opens on to the surface at the **sacral hiatus** where the posterior part of the vertebral arch remains deficient throughout life. In life this is closed with a little loose fibrous tissue. Lateral to this midline crest on either side is the so-called **articular crest.** These represent the fused articular processes of the sacral vertebrae. The four posterior sacral foramina transmit the dorsal rami. The 5th sacral foramina is formed on either side of the sacral hiatus. From it emerge the small 5th sacral nerve and coccygeal nerves. Lateral to these foramina a lateral crest represents the fused transverse processes of the sacral vertebrae.

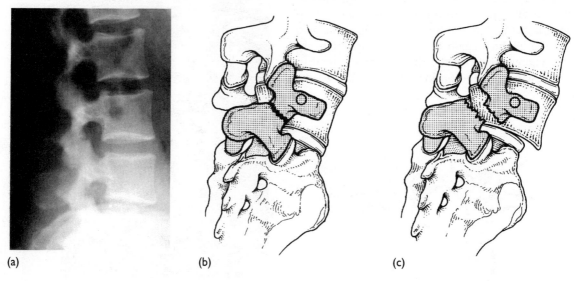

(a)   (b)   (c)

Figure 13.24   (a) Lateral radiograph of the lumbar region. Note that the boundaries of an intervertebral foramen are the bodies and disc anteriorly, the pedicles above and below, and the synovial facet joints posteriorly. (b) Tracing of an oblique radiograph view of the lumbar column. Understand how in an actual radiograph the nose of the 'Scottie dog' is the transverse process, the eye is a pedicle and the ear is a superior articular process. The neck and collar lie between the superior and inferior articular processes. This region is called the pars interarticularis. A radiolucent pars is either fractured or cartilaginous. (c) Bilateral fracture of both pars, or bilateral congenitally unfused pars, results in **spondylolisthesis.** Here the body of L5 has shifted forwards on the sacrum. ((b) and (c) after Keim, HA and Kirkaldy-Willis, WH (1980) Low back pain. *Clinical Symposia* **32**(6).)

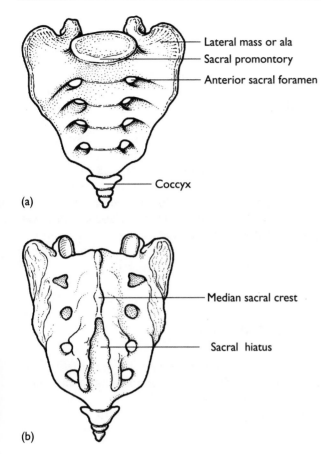

(a)

(b)

Figure 13.25 The sacrum and coccyx seen (a) from the front and (b) from behind.

There are sex differences between the male and female sacrum. The most notable of these is apparent when the width of the body of the 1st of the first sacral segment and the width of its lateral mass are compared (Fig. 13.26). The sacrum as a whole is wider in the female and the body narrower.

Local anaesthetic can be introduced into the extra-dural space by passing a needle into the region of the sacral hiatus. Anaesthesia of the lower sacral and coccygeal nerves is useful in obstetric procedures on the vagina. The coccyx is all that is left of the tail. In humans it is represented by four small fused bones. It is joined to the apex of the sacrum by an intervertebral disc and laterally by two small synovial joints.

The contents of the vertebral canal

The vertebral canal is a smooth-walled tube in which the spinal cord lies. It is lined in front by the posterior longitudinal ligament which covers the vertebral bodies and discs. Behind it is lined with the ligamentum flavum, which joins adjacent laminae. Above it is continuous with the cranial cavity through the foramen magnum in the base of the skull. Here, the spinal cord is continuous above with the brain. The lower end of the canal is open through the small sacral hiatus at the lower end of the sacrum. The only other openings in the tube are the pairs of intervertebral foramina that are found at each intervertebral level.

On opening the vertebral canal, the first obvious thing one sees is a collection of loose fat. Through this fat the vertebral and spinal veins and arteries pass. On removing the fat the membranous coverings of the spinal cord become visible and inside these is the cord itself. The extradural fat of the vertebral canal contains a rich plexus of veins. The whole network, which runs longitudinally through the entire length of the canal, is called the **internal vertebral venous plexus** (Fig. 13.27).

Blood drains into this plexus from both the spinal cord and the vertebral bodies. The vertebral body of

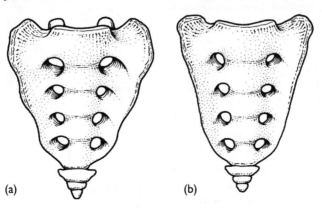

(a)   (b)

Figure 13.26 The sacrum in the female (a) is proportioned differently to that in the male (b). (See text.)

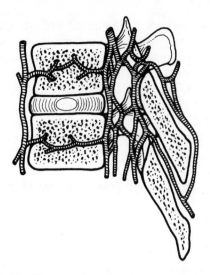

Figure 13.27   The extradural fat within the spinal canal contains a rich plexus of veins called the internal vertebral venous plexus. This plexus communicates with veins in the vertebral bodies and in the abdomen, and with the external vertebral venous plexus.

each vertebra contains erythropoietic bone marrow. It must therefore have good venous drainage to take newly formed red blood cells into the circulation. Usually there are two **basivertebral veins** leaving each body. All of the veins in this plexus are valveless and so blood can travel in any direction through them. The internal vertebral venous plexus drains through each intervertebral foramen to connect with the **external vertebral venous plexus** which is found surrounding the entire vertebral column. Much of this plexus lies in the muscle masses found at the back and in front of the column. Eventually, all this network of blood vessels drains into the segmental veins of the body wall. In the thoracic region this means the posterior intercostal veins; in the abdomen, the lumbar veins. Since the vertebral venous plexuses are valveless, reverse flow occurs easily. This happens, for example, when coughing and sneezing or during prolonged periods of raised intrathoracic and intra-abdominal pressure, such as during childbirth or when lifting heavy loads. Blood is momentarily diverted to the vertebral venous plexus and then later finds its way back through either the intercostal veins or lumbar veins into the superior and inferior vena cava. During all this, the pressure in the vertebral column rises. Cancer cells can spread easily between the abdomen and thorax through this sort of retrograde

venous flow, and so commonly come to lodge in the vertebral bodies.

The spinal cord is supplied with arterial blood mainly from above (Fig. 13.28). An **anterior** and two **posterior spinal arteries** arise from the vertebral artery in the region of the foramen magnum. The anterior artery descends in the midline groove on the spinal cord. The two posterior vessels pass down the posterior surface of the cord. At each spinal segment, however, these arteries are reinforced by segmental spinal arteries. These vessels are branches of body wall segmental arteries. In the thoracic region this would be the intercostal arteries. These are, however, mostly fairly small except at the 1st and 11th thoracic segments. Each artery enters the vertebral canal through the intervertebral foramen.

The meninges

When the fat and plexuses of veins and arteries have been removed from the vertebral canal a clear view is obtained of the spinal cord and its coverings. Both brain and spinal cord are covered with a continuous, three-layered protective sleeve called the meninges

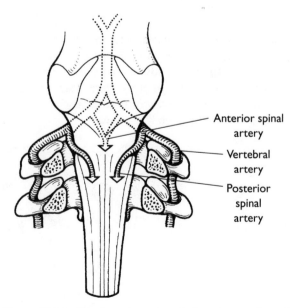

Anterior spinal artery

Vertebral artery

Posterior spinal artery

Figure 13.28   Blood supply to the spinal cord comes from the anterior and posterior spinal arteries which are reinforced at each spinal segmental level via spinal arteries.

(Fig. 13.29). The inner layer of this sleeve is a delicate membrane closely applied to the surface of the neuraxis. It is called the **pia mater**. It dips into the fissures and indentations of the brain and spinal cord, and in it run many small blood vessels on their way to supply nervous tissue.

The middle layer is the **arachnoid mater**. It does not closely invest the brain and spinal cord, such that it encloses a space between the arachnoid and pial layers. This space is called the **subarachnoid space**. The space is not empty, but contains fluid called the **cerebrospinal fluid** (CSF). This fluid acts as a buffer and shock absorber, so protecting the nervous tissue from trauma. It is produced in the cavities of the brain. It circulates in the subarachnoid space surrounding the whole neuraxis, and it is then absorbed into the venous blood via **arachnoid granulations** which are found in some of the venous sinuses of the cranial cavity. There is therefore a 'circulation' of CSF: production in the cavities of the brain, circulation through the subarachnoid space and absorption into the venous blood in the cranial cavity. The arachnoid sends fine web-like processes through the CSF to attach to the pia. In certain parts of the skull and vertebral canal the subarachnoid space is enlarged. These pools of CSF are called cisterns.

The arachnoid lies beneath the outer layer of meninges called the **dura mater**. There is only a capillary interval between the two. This is the subdural space. The dura mater is thick, fibrous and strong. In certain places in the skull it is fused to the periosteum of the bone. In other places there is a gap between the dura and periosteum. These gaps are filled with venous blood. They are called the **cranial venous sinuses** (Fig. 13.30). It will be seen from Figure 13.30 that the dural sheath of the brain is directly continuous with that of the spinal cord, and both cranial venous sinuses and internal vertebral venous plexuses lie within the extradural space.

In the vertebral canal, the dura forms a kind of tube. It is not fused to the periosteum of the vertebra but is separated from the walls of the canal by extradural fat and vessels. The space between the dura and the bony walls is called the extradural space. Along all the segmental spinal nerves the dura is drawn out with them into the intervertebral foramina. The attachments to the intervertebral foramina act to stabilize the dural tube in the vertebral canal.

The spinal cord, lying in this tube of dura and arachnoid, is in addition buffered against shocks by the CSF. Small tooth-like processes of pia mater arise from each side of the spinal cord. These arise from the pia between dorsal and ventral roots. They pass through the CSF and pierce the arachnoid to gain attachment to the dura. They therefore suspend the cord from the dural tube. They are called the **ligamenta denticulata**. The lowest ligamentum denticulatum is found at the level of the 1st lumbar roots (Fig. 13.31).

The spinal cord itself is about 18 inches long in

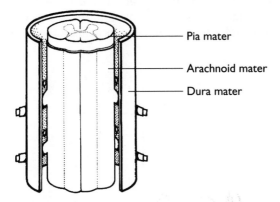

Figure 13.29 Three layers of meninges surround the brain and spinal cord. The pia mater is inextricably associated with the surface of the brain and spinal cord. The arachnoid encloses a space between itself and the pia, called the subarachnoid space, which is full of CSF. The dura is thick and tough. In fact, there is only a capillary interval between the arachnoid and the dura.

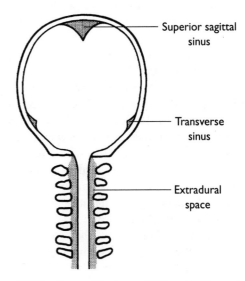

Figure 13.30 Dura within the skull is fused to the periosteum except where cranial venous sinuses run between the two. Within the vertebral canal the dura is separated from the bony walls by extradural fat containing the internal vertebral venous plexus.

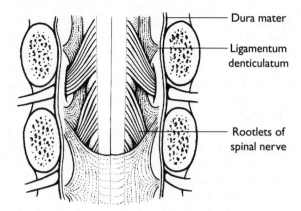

Dura mater

Ligamentum
denticulatum

Rootlets of
spinal nerve

Figure 13.31   Between the ventral and dorsal rootlets of the spinal cord, tooth-like projections of pia mater arise. They pass through the CSF and pierce the arachnoid to anchor to the dura at the sides. These are the ligamenta denticulata, which suspend the spinal cord from the dura mater.

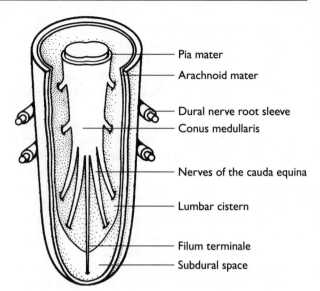

Pia mater

Arachnoid mater

Dural nerve root sleeve

Conus medullaris

Nerves of the cauda equina

Lumbar cistern

Filum terminale

Subdural space

Figure 13.32   In the adult, the conus medullaris ends at the level of L1 or L2. The arachnoid and dura extend beyond this to the level of S2. The filum terminale is an extension of pia mater and fibrous tissue. It extends down to the end of the sacrum and is fixed to the second coccygeal segment.

adults. It does not extend to the end of the vertebral canal but reaches down only to about the lower border of the 2nd lumbar vertebra. This is not so at birth. Here the cord extends much lower but, as the vertebral column grows at a greater rate, it draws away from the cord leaving it positioned progressively higher up in the canal. The roots of the spinal nerves therefore need to run further to their intervertebral foramina. This is especially true of the lower lumbar and sacral roots.

The arrangements of the cord and meninges at the lower end of the vertebral column needs special attention (Fig. 13.32). The spinal cord and its covering of pia end at about the level of the lower border of the 2nd lumbar vertebra. However, a thin strand of pia called the **filum terminale** continues down through the subarachnoid space into the sacral part of the canal. Here it pierces the dura and is attached near the sacral hiatus. Its function is similar to that of the ligamentum denticulatum in that it helps to suspend the cord in the CSF. The dura and arachnoid do not end with the cord and pia either. They continue down to the level of the 2nd sacral segment. Hence, there is a large subarachnoid space in this region called the **lumbar cistern**. The roots of the lumbar and sacral nerves run through this cistern. They look like a horse's tail and so have been named the **cauda equina**.

Applied anatomy of the vertebral canal

The lumbar cistern is a convenient place to remove CSF for clinical analysis. The procedure is called **lumbar puncture** (Figs 13.33 and 13.34). The patient's back is marked with two lines. One is a vertical midline and the other is horizontal, joining the two iliac crests. The horizontal line marks the 4th lumbar spine in the midline. A sterile needle is introduced between the 4th and 5th spines under a local anaesthetic. This

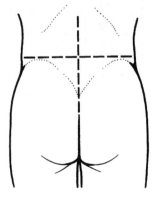

Figure 13.33   The 4th lumbar spine lies in the midline on a line joining the top of the two iliac crests.

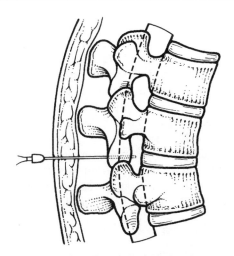

Figure 13.34   A needle passed between the 4th and 5th lumbar spines passes through the supraspinous and interspinous ligaments, then the ligamentum flavum and extradural fat. The dura may offer some resistance before it then passes through it and the arachnoid mater, and finally into the CSF within the subarachnoid space.

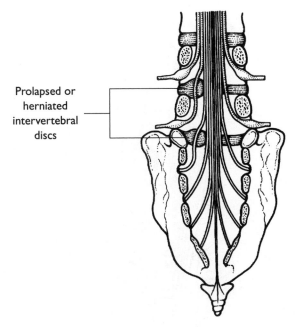

Prolapsed or herniated intervertebral discs

Figure 13.35   Prolapsed intervertebral discs between L4 and L5 and between L5 and S1 are pressing here on segmental nerves L5 and S1. Understand how discs that prolapse nearer the midline at these levels can affect nerve roots that exit lower down in the sacrum.

level is well below the termination of the spinal cord and so the needle can safely be introduced further into the subarachnoid space. CSF can then be aspirated. No damage to the nerve roots occurs since they float away from the needle in the pool of CSF. Not only can a specimen of CSF be taken, but the pressure of the CSF can also be measured. Normally it is 60–200 mm of CSF. Coughing and sneezing increase this pressure due to the increase in blood flow through the vertebral venous plexuses. Similarly, radio-opaque dye can be injected into the subarachnoid space. In this way tumours of the cord may be explored by radiograph investigation; this procedure is called **myelography**.

Figure 13.35 illustrates two 'slipped discs' at the level of the intervertebral discs between L4 and L5 and between L5 and the sacrum. Here, the nucleus pulposus has protruded through the tough annulus fibrosus and is now exerting pressure on nerve roots L5 and S1. It is not difficult to see how easily this can cause pain and sensory loss in the lower limb as well as wasting of the leg muscles on occasions. 'Slipped discs' and 'sciatica' are extremely common complaints.

The musculature of the vertebral column

The vertebral column is surrounded by muscles. In places this is very thick and strong whilst in others it is weak or even absent. The musculature of the body wall is composed of three layers. Often muscles migrate during development in order to serve different functions. However, a general rule still holds in that the **internal layer** lies inside the ribs or costal elements of the vertebrae, the **middle layer** lies between costal elements or ribs and the **outer layer** lies outside them. There are two good examples of muscles derived from the inner layer that are closely associated with the vertebral column. The **prevertebral muscles** in the cervical and thoracic regions and the **psoas major** in the lumbar region of the vertebral column (Fig. 13.36). The origins and insertions of these muscles are from vertebral bodies and discs, and they are supplied by ventral rami of appropriate spinal nerves.

Examples of muscles that are derived from the middle layer in the region of the vertebral column are the **scalene muscles** in the neck and the **quadratus**

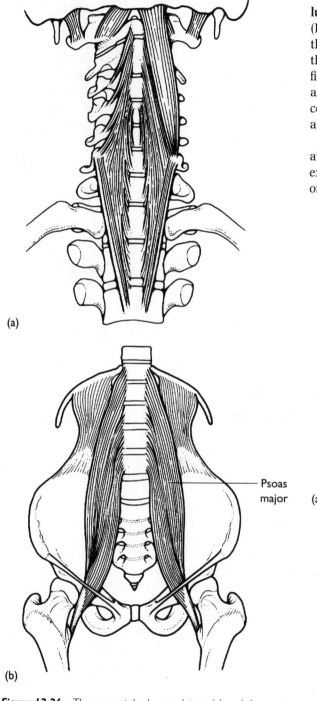

(a)

(b)

Figure 13.36 The prevertebral musculature (a) and the psoas muscle (b) are examples of muscles that originate inside the ribs or costal elements of the vertebrae.

lumborum in the lumbar region of the column (Fig. 13.37). The scalene muscles arise in part from the anterior tubercles of certain cervical vertebrae, that is from the costal elements, and insert into the first two ribs. Similarly, the quadratus lumborum arises from the ilium and inserts into transverse processes of the lumbar vertebrae (both costal elements) and into the 12th rib.

The third layer or external group of muscles associated with the vertebral column is very strong and extends on either side from the sacrum up to the base of the skull. They may be collectively called the **erec-**

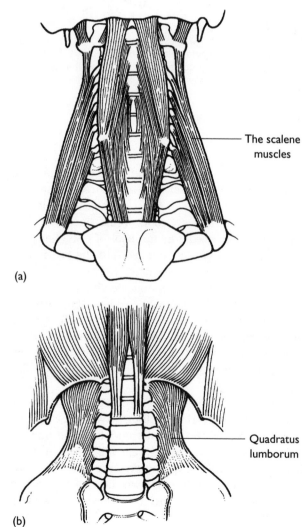

The scalene muscles

(a)

Quadratus lumborum

(b)

Figure 13.37 The scalene muscles (a) and the quadratus lumborum (b) are examples of muscles that originate between costal elements of vertebrae or ribs.

tor spinae mass. They are the only muscles in the body supplied by **dorsal rami** of the spinal nerves.

There is little value in remembering the names of the individual bundles of muscle fibres in the erector spinae mass. However, a few basic concepts are useful since fibres of these muscles, as well as the small ligaments uniting vertebrae, are frequently the cause of recurrent back problems.

The erector spinae mass is divided into two main muscle groups, the **sacrospinalis** and the **transverse** spinalis group. The sacrospinalis group is composed of three muscle sets which extend from the sacrum to the skull and which lie vertically (Fig. 13.38). In the lowermost part the muscle arises from the back of the sacrum and is covered with a strong aponeurosis. The transverse spinalis group is also composed of three sets of muscle, but these lie one on top of the other in the groove between the spines and transverse processes of the vertebrae. All these small muscle groups arise laterally from parts of the vertebral arch

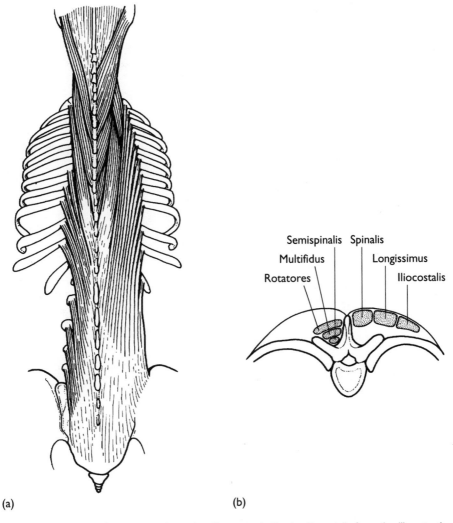

(a)   (b)

Figure 13.38 The superficial sacrospinalis group of muscles all run vertically: the iliocostalis from the ilium to the ribs, the longissimus group between the transverse processes of the vertebrae, and the spinalis group between the spines of the vertebrae of the thoracic and lumbar regions. The deeper transverse spinalis group of muscles all run obliquely from a lateral attachment on to the transverse process of a vertebra to the midline spinous process of another vertebra. The deepest rotatores muscle bundles run the entire length of the column in short spans between each adjacent vertebra. The multifidus bundles also run the entire length of the column but in spans of two to five vertebrae. The semispinalis run only from T10 upwards. All these muscles together are known as the **intrinsic muscles of the back.**

and proceed medially to insert into the spinous processes (Fig. 13.38). The erector spinae group **extends** the vertebral column. These movements are marked in the lumbar and cervical regions. The smaller deeper group of the muscle mass is also able to make fine adjusting movements which include rotation of one vertebra on another. **Flexion** of the vertebral column is produced by such muscles as the prevertebral and psoas muscles. Lateral flexion in the lumbar region is effected by the quadratus lumborum muscle.

chapter
14

Revision of the Vertebral Column and Spinal Canal

Use the following multiple choice questions to assess your knowledge of the vertebral column and spinal canal. Remember, any of the options A–E may be correct or incorrect. After you have attempted them all, refer back to the text if you need assistance with any of the options. Once again a score of around 50% at your first attempt would be acceptable.

Multiple Choice Questions on the Vertebral Column

1. Concerning the cervical part of the vertebral column:
(A) there are eight cervical vertebrae
(B) the 1st cervical vertebra possesses no body
(C) typical cervical vertebrae have a bifid spinous process
(D) the 7th cervical vertebra is called the vertebra prominens
(E) cervical vertebrae have a large triangular vertebral canal

A____ B ____ C ____ D ___ E ____

2. The atlas:
(A) has two foramina transversaria
(B) has a bifid spinous process
(C) articulates with the dens at a fibrous joint
(D) articulates with superior articular facets on the axis
(E) has uncinate processes

A____ B ____ C ____ D ___ E ____

3. The second cervical vertebra or axis:
(A) has no spinous process
(B) has no body
(C) transmits the weight of the head through the dens
(D) has flat superior articular facets above for articulation with the atlas
(E) has the vertebral artery passing posteriorly behind its lateral mass

A____ B ____ C ____ D ____ E ____

4. Typical thoracic vertebrae:
(A) have long spinous processes that project inferiorly
(B) have facet joints that allow considerable flexion and extension
(C) have transverse processs that form synovial joints with ribs
(D) have superior and inferior hemifacets that form synovial joints with ribs
(E) have intervertebral foramina that can be seen on a lateral radiograph of the chest

A____ B ____ C ____ D ___ E ____

5. Typical lumbar vertebrae:
(A) have large kidney-shaped bodies
(B) have smaller vertebral foramina than cervical vertebrae
(C) have longer spinous processes than thoracic vertebrae
(D) have a 'pars interarticularis' visible on oblique radiograph between the superior and inferior articular facets
(E) allow extensive rotational movements in the lumbar region

A____ B ____ C ____ D ____ E ____

6. The boundaries of an intervertebral foramen in the lumbar region include:
(A) the anterior longitudinal ligament
(B) the pedicles of two vertebrae
(C) the spinous process
(D) the annulus fibrosus
(E) a facet joint

A____ B ____ C ____ D ___ E ____

7. The sacrum:

(A) contains the terminal portion of the spinal cord at birth
(B) is composed of four fused sacral segments
(C) forms a secondary cartilaginous joint with the ilium
(D) is proportioned differently in men and women
(E) is always deficient in the midline posteriorly over the last fused segment

A____ B ____ C ____ D ____ E ____

8. The internal vertebral venous plexus:

(A) has valves
(B) is found in the extradural space (epidural space) of the vertebral canal
(C) receives basivertebral veins
(D) receives veins that pass through the intervertebral foramina
(E) communicates with the external vertebral venous plexus

A____ B ____ C ____ D ____ E ____

9. The following structures are composed solely of pia mater:

(A) the cauda equina
(B) the conus medullaris
(C) the filum terminale
(D) a ligamentum denticulatum
(E) ligamentum flavum

A____ B ____ C ____ D ____ E ____

10. A lumbar puncture needle passing into the subarachnoid space should pierce:

(A) the membranous layer of superficial fascia (Scarpa)
(B) the space between the 4th and 5th lumbar spinous processes
(C) extradural (epidural) fat
(D) the pia
(E) the dura and arachnoid

A____ B ____ C ____ D ____ E ____

Answers to Multiple Choice Questions

1.	AF	BT	CT	DT	ET
2.	AT	BF	CF	DT	EF
3.	AF	BF	CF	DT	EF
4.	AT	BF	CT	DT	ET

5.	AT	BT	CF	DT	EF
6.	AF	BT	CF	DT	ET
7.	AF	BF	CF	DT	ET

8.	AF	BT	CT	DT	ET
9.	AF	BF	CT	DT	EF
10.	AF	BT	CT	DF	ET

Index

Numbers in *italics* refer to illustrations